Praise for
The Satisfied Guide to Eating Well

"In *The Satisfied Guide to Eating Well*, Dr. Rhona Epstein shares an important message about food addiction that is missing from too many eating disorder programs—addiction is a brain disorder. This book helps you find ways to rewire your brain to help you gain control over food and your life."

—Daniel G. Amen, MD, author of
Change Your Brain Every Day

"*The Satisfied Guide to Eating Well* is a well-established approach for overcoming addictive eating habits based on science, tradition, and expertise of both nutrition and addiction. This will be a valuable resource for anyone seeking to improve an addictive relationship with food and particularly helpful for the person who is ready for recovery."

—David Wiss, PhD, MS, RDN,
founder of Nutrition in Recovery

"Dr. Rhona Epstein is a leading expert and trusted voice on food addiction recovery from a biblical perspective. *The Satisfied Guide to Eating Well* is packed full of real wisdom and practical guidance offering a comprehensive approach to overcoming unhealthy eating behaviors by creating thoughtful food plans. This resource book recognizes that the journey to wellness is as much mental, emotional, and spiritual as it is physical."

—Tim Clinton, EdD, LPC, LMFT, president of
the American Association of Christian Counselors
and executive director of the Liberty University
Global Center for Human Flourishing

Praise for Dr. Rhona's *Food Triggers*

"A masterpiece of a roadmap designed to bring love, acceptance, freedom, and, most of all, balance back into the lives of those torn up by the claws of addictions."

—Lindsay Roberts, author, speaker, and co-host of *The Place for Miracles* and host of *Make Your Day Count*

"Dr. Rhona has the unique and potent combination of her personal recovery experience as well as professional training to help those still suffering. Her book brings to life what food addiction is, the research that substantiates it, and hope for anyone still suffering. There is a way to freedom!"

—Kim Dennis, MD, CEDS, co-founder, CEO, and chief medical officer at SunCloud Health and former CEO and medical director at Timberline Knolls

THE *Satisfied*
GUIDE TO EATING WELL

THE
Satisfied
GUIDE TO EATING WELL

Dr. Rhona Epstein, PSY.D
with Jackie Mack, MS, RDN, LDN

A HEALTHY PLAN FOR
Your Spiritual Journey
TOWARD FOOD FREEDOM

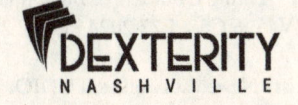

DEXTERITY
NASHVILLE

DEXTERITY

604 Magnolia Lane
Nashville, TN 37211

Copyright © 2024 by Rhona Epstein.

Scripture quotations marked NKJV are taken from New King James Version®. Copyright © 1982 by Thomas Nelson. Used by permission. All rights reserved.

Scripture quotations marked ESV are taken from the ESV® Bible (The Holy Bible, English Standard Version®). Copyright © 2001 by Crossway, a publishing ministry of Good News Publishers. Used by permission. All rights reserved.

All rights reserved. Except as permitted by the US Copyright Act of 1976, no part of this book may be reproduced, distributed, or transmitted without prior written permission from the publisher. For information, please contact info@dexteritybooks.com.

Printed in the United States of America.

First edition: 2024
10 9 8 7 6 5 4 3 2 1

ISBN: 978-1-947297-94-4 (Trade Paperback)
ISBN: 978-1-947297-94-4 (E-book)

Publisher's Cataloging-in-Publication Data:

Names: Epstein, Rhona, author. | Mack, Jackie, author.
Title: The satisfied guide to eating well / Dr. Rhona Epstein, PSY.D; with Jackie Mack, MS, RDN, LDN.
Description: Includes bibliographical references. | Nashville, TN: Dexterity, 2024.
Identifiers: ISBN: 978-1-947297-94-4 (paperback) | 978-1-947297-95-1 (e-book)
Subjects: LCSH Food--Religious aspects--Christianity. | Compulsive eating---Religious aspects--Christianity. | Compulsive eating--Psychological aspects. | Compulsive eaters--Rehabilitation. | Spirituality. | BISAC RELIGION / Christian Living / Personal Growth | COOKING / Health & Healing / General | SELF-HELP / Eating Disorders & Body Image
Classification: LCC BV4596.C58 .E77 2024 | DDC 261.8/3225--dc23

Cover design by Charissa Newell at twolineSTUDIO.
Interior design by PerfecType.

A NOTE TO THE READER

This book was created with the intention of providing general nutrition education. The information shared is based on scientifically supported evidence and is aligned with the recommended standards for food and nutrition in the United States of America.

Prior to implementing any kind of dietary, supplemental, or behavioral lifestyle changes, please consult your physician and/or medical team to ensure this is the right decision for you. Please do not make any changes or discontinue any prescribed medical treatment based on the content of this book.

The goal is to provide insight into how to live a healthy lifestyle through an open-structured format while emphasizing food, nutrition, and generalized wellness. In order to successfully tailor the program to your individual needs, it is recommended that you schedule a meeting with a licensed dietitian who specializes in food addiction.

Dedication

To the precious people suffering in the throes of addictive eating and food obsession—may you find peace and freedom!

CONTENTS

Introduction: Dr. Rhona's Story xiii

Part I: Diagnose the Problem

Chapter 1: So How Do I Start? 3
Chapter 2: Sugar Addiction 23
Chapter 3: Approaching Your Food Plan—It's All About Mindset 35
Chapter 4: Emotional Eating 47
Chapter 5: Spirituality 55
Chapter 6: Habits 61
Chapter 7: Planning and Preparing—Give Up Excuses and Make Up Your Mind 69
Chapter 8: Backup Plans—Restaurants and Vacations 81
Chapter 9: Parties, Holidays, and Catered Affairs 93

Part II: Pick Your Path

Chapter 10: Narrowing It Down 107
Chapter 11: The Building Blocks of Nutrition 125
Chapter 12: Food Planning 145

Chapter 13: Food Plan Examples	163
Chapter 14: Commonly Asked Questions	175

Part III: Transform Your Mealtimes

Breakfast Recipes	188
Lunch Recipes	201
Dinner Recipes	216
Side Dish Recipes	236
Dressing Recipes	242
Snack Recipes	245
Holiday Recipes	248
Dr. Rhona's Food Freedom Tips	254
Acknowledgments	257
Appendix: Additional Food Plans	259
Notes	265
About the Authors	269

INTRODUCTION

Dr. Rhona's Story

If you picked up this book, I'm guessing you have a troubled (maybe even tormented) relationship with food and eating.

You are not alone.

Growing up, I always had a problem with food. I abused food as a kid well into my teens, and I was completely and totally hooked on sugar, white flour, and highly processed foods. I'm not exaggerating when I say the only foods I ate were what tasted good: pasta, cake, cookies, ice cream, pizza. If it was bad for me, I couldn't get enough of it. My daily meal intake looked like a box of Cap'n Crunch® or Pop-Tarts® in the morning for breakfast, peanut butter and jelly sandwiches on white bread for lunch, and noodles for dinner.

I would consume half gallons of ice cream in one sitting, entire boxes of Oreo® cookies, whole jars of peanut butter. I was going for the highest intensity of sugar I could get my

INTRODUCTION

hands on. All I thought about was the next time I could find something sweeter.

By the time I was twelve, I was out of control: bulimic, abusing diet pills, constantly trying to lose weight with crazy fad diets, starving myself during the day, and bingeing and purging well into the night. I tried any new diet I could get my hands on, no matter how off-the-wall it sounded. If something promised it could get me to lose weight, I would try it—but nothing worked. I was completely consumed by my toxic relationship with food.

Of course, at the time, I didn't know it was toxic. I also didn't know that the main reason I was turning to food was for comfort. I grew up in a home where I felt emotionally unsupported. My mother was critical and rejecting, and I felt totally unloved by her. These intense feelings of rejection resulted in insecurity, self-consciousness, and self-hate.

On the other hand, I was close with my dad, and one of the main ways we connected was through eating. It sounds extreme, but some of the only times I felt truly loved in my childhood were when my dad took me to Baskin-Robbins and we ate ice cream together. That was how we connected. The food provided a feeling of camaraderie, and I was desperate for any kind of parental love or acceptance in the emotional wake my mother left. Eating ice cream with my dad was love; therefore, *food* was love. The combination of bonding over food

INTRODUCTION

with my dad to feel loved and turning to food for comfort from my mother's emotional rejection set the stage for a confusing relationship with food—both charged and contradictory.

In my house growing up, there was a lot of confusion and mixed messages. Our house was chock-full of treats and junk food, but I was simultaneously criticized by my mother when I ate any of it. She deeply shamed me for my weight, and the expectation was that I should be thin, despite our house having almost no nourishing food in sight. My mother criticized me constantly, looking at me in disgust because I was gaining weight. But food was my place for comfort, and it's exactly where I went whenever she made those disparaging comments. It was absolutely crazy-making; I couldn't win, no matter what I did. I didn't understand any of what was happening to me until I was much older—but we'll get to that.

Things started escalating around the time I turned twelve. My mother initiated me into the dieting world, and this created a whole other layer of insanity for me. I wasn't desperate to connect with Mom; I was trying to get as far away from her and her criticism as I possibly could. But she was invested in getting me thin and I wanted that too. This, of course, did not end well. It wasn't long before the hiding, lying, and sneaking began. I was secretly bingeing, ravenous after not eating all day. I would lie to my mother when she asked why I was gaining weight, making up whatever excuses I could to

INTRODUCTION

cover my out-of-control appetite and behavior. My life was a mess that I was desperate to control—even though, at twelve, I obviously had no way of doing that. The worst part was I felt so incredibly isolated in my pain and suffering.

I grew up in the '70s, when the notion of "eating disorders" was nowhere to be seen in public consciousness. Sure, it was important to some of my friends to be thin, but I didn't know *anyone* who felt about food the way I did, and no one was using words like *bulimia* or *eating disorder*. Food was on my mind all day, every day. Either I was eating it or I was obsessing about *not* eating it—stuck in an endless thought loop of what I would eat next and then what I would have to do to get rid of it. I was completely adrift and I felt like I was losing my mind. I was absolutely hijacked by this obsession, and it was ruining my life.

I tried everything to get this madness to stop. As I said, I went on every single diet under the sun but couldn't follow any of them. I begged my parents to put locks on the freezer doors and the cabinets, but after they did, I found a way to open them anyway.

For most of my teenage years, I was overweight, yes, and obsessed, yes. Extreme dieting and exercising kept my weight from creeping up too high. However, around sixteen or seventeen, my toxic habits became more visible. I'd down a dozen donuts on a thirty-minute drive or get up in the middle

INTRODUCTION

of the night to empty the pantry's stock of peanut butter, and my insane dieting measures could no longer keep up. To give you an idea of how depraved my thinking had become, I began to fantasize about moving to another country, one where it was "acceptable" to be overweight. I couldn't see any way I would ever be thin, and that felt overwhelming.

Again, in the 1970s there was little understanding of eating disorders—no treatment centers, no "eating disorder" diagnoses. It was incredibly isolating being in the midst of something no one was talking about. I had no peace—though I was absolutely desperate for it—and began to feel that something was deeply and fundamentally wrong with me. All I wanted to do was eat donuts and Rocky Road ice cream, but at the same time, I would have given *anything* to figure out how to stop.

This was my rock bottom. I fell into a severe depression, thick in a fog of self-hate, insecurity, drug abuse, suicidal thinking, pulling away from my friends, and hanging out with people I knew were bad news. I thought about dying every single day. At this time, I was taking amphetamines and other pills and smoking marijuana, desperate for anything to curb my appetite, only to inevitably binge on bags of chips and boxes of cookies once I crashed.

I was doing terribly in school; I couldn't pay attention in class, let alone complete my homework. I would later learn

INTRODUCTION

that sugar has this effect on the brain: causing focus issues, disordered thinking, and more. Since I was literally only eating foods containing insanely high amounts of sugar, it's no wonder I felt like I was going out of my mind. I was a zombie, and the only thing keeping me alive was dreaming of a different life, free of my impossible problem.

A FLICKER OF HOPE

In the throes of this desperation at age seventeen, at my lowest point, I ran into an acquaintance I had met while working at a summer camp. Some time had passed since I'd last seen him, and I couldn't help but notice he had lost a lot of weight. More than that, though, something was different about him. He seemed lighter, self-assured, and more importantly, free. I could tell he had been transformed in some way. I was at the point in my obsession where I truly wished I could die; I was so sick of the torment, so tired of the endless, exhausting spiral of my own behavior and patterns. Whatever it was that he had, I wanted some of it—and not just because he had clearly lost weight.

Something in me was stirred to ask him about his transformation: what had happened in his life for him to so obviously have changed? For the record, this was *totally* unlike me at the time. My shame and anxiety often manifested in shyness and awkwardness, especially when it came to personal matters. I can only attribute the reason for my asking to God; I truly believe that my conversation with this young man I barely knew was a divine appointment.

He told me that he had begun going to a support group nearby since the last time we'd seen each other, and he described a group of people who met weekly to discuss their problems with food. He told me the location of one of the meetings and gently encouraged me to go. That was one of the most important moments of my whole life, because it introduced me to the recovery process.

The following week, I attended my first meeting. It is not an exaggeration to say that going to this meeting changed my life. The moment people began to share, it became clear to me that I wasn't the only person in the world dealing with the feelings and experiences that I believed were ruining my life. Person after person spoke of their own journeys, and they could have been reading pages from my diary. It is one of the first times in my life I felt truly understood, and definitely the first moment in my life when I sensed a flicker of hope that freedom from the insanity might be possible. There was such power in hearing these stories told out loud, with absolutely no judgment from the people listening.

During any given meeting of this support group, people gathered for one hour, sharing their experiences of overeating

INTRODUCTION

or abusing food, supplemented with readings from what's called the "Big Book"—aka, the manual for alcoholics, originally written by Alcoholics Anonymous founder Bill W. This was the first time I had ever been exposed to the idea that certain foods and the behaviors attached to them were akin to alcoholism. This was a total revelation: the way I was living, the ways I thought about food, were as detrimental as the behaviors and thinking of someone struggling with alcoholism. This was groundbreaking.

This place had nothing to do with fad diets or crazy exercise routines. It was clear that the philosophy of the group was to identify with one another's mutual inability to control something that was clearly out of control. Members called their behaviors "insanity," and boy, did that resonate. The simplicity of hearing people share their stories out loud, in front of other people, made me realize on a cellular level that I wasn't alone. The literature used in these meetings from the Big Book was the first time I heard the vocabulary to articulate to myself what I was actually experiencing. This language of addiction got through to me like no diet or philosophy ever had.

My name is Rhona, and I am a compulsive overeater.

All these years later, I can still remember one of the stories someone told that first day: how they had "officially sworn off this junk food item for good," only to find themselves digging through the trash for it hours later. I had done the exact same

INTRODUCTION

thing. These people truly understood how I was feeling, and it was the first time I dared to hope there was a cure.

YOU ARE NOT ALONE

Even though I felt seen and understood by these people, I wasn't hooked on the support group right away. As I mentioned, I was a teenager, and most of the people there were older than me, which felt off-putting. (Now, though, I view this as one of the great strengths of support groups: you can learn from anyone, especially someone you view as "different from you.") Sure, they described exactly what I was going through, but I didn't see myself coming back. I was too depressed to really think straight, even after seeing a ray of light.

One young woman in the group was a few years older than me, and she sought me out after that first meeting. She could tell I was hesitant, so she asked for my number and later called to persuade me to come back. She said that she had seen me at the local Y a few times, running on the indoor track for an hour and then swimming for miles, trying to get rid of my binge eating weight. She encouraged me that I didn't have to live like that anymore, that there was hope for someone like me if I came back.

I did eventually get hooked on the process (at last, hooked on something good for me), but it took the encouragement of someone who had been there before and could see just a little further ahead on the path. It's not an exaggeration to say I owe my recovery to that young woman.

FINDING MY PURPOSE IN HELPING OTHERS

During my many years battling food addiction, I so longed for somebody to turn to for help. The recovery group changed my life. I knew that once I was firmly established in the recovery process, I wanted to spend my life doing the same thing for others.

I began working with drug addicts and alcoholics in the early '80s, noticing the similarities between those addictions and food addiction, although food addiction was still controversial and wasn't considered in the mainstream. The only people I encountered who understood the ins and outs of food addiction were people in 12-step recovery themselves, regardless of which program. When I was in my twenties, there was still so much resistance—both in the cultural conversation and among psychological and medical professionals—to the idea that food could be as addictive for some people as any drug.

While there is still room for improvement, so much has changed. There are all kinds of recovery groups available for food addicts, along with research to support how sugar is both highly addictive and can change your brain chemistry (we'll

INTRODUCTION

get into that later in the book). Professionals across disciplines, from social workers to therapists to nutritionists, recognize this addiction as something treatable. I personally believe we are closer than ever to getting a food addiction diagnosis in the *Diagnostic and Statistical Manual of Mental Disorders* (DSM).

Because of my own experiences, I have been able to be part of this movement from the ground up. It hasn't been easy; in fact, it has been an uphill battle getting others in the psychology field to take this health issue seriously. Whenever I feel frustrated or discouraged, I return to the memory of that first recovery meeting. I remember what it felt like to feel hopeless, only to find out there *was* hope. I completely get why people have a hard time understanding food addiction; it's incredibly difficult to wrap your head around it if you haven't been there.

And so I keep doing my best to push this conversation forward. I share all this with you in hopes of imparting what was imparted to me in that first support group meeting: *you are not alone.* If my work helps just one person feel that they're not abandoned and that there is an alternative of freedom to the way they are living, it will have been worth it. If any of what I've shared in these first few pages reflects your own experience, you are in the right place.

I can help you, because I've been where you are. I know what it's like to feel like there's no "out," that life isn't worth

INTRODUCTION

living, and that you're losing your mind. I know what it's like to feel scared, hopeless, and depressed, with no place to turn. For some readers, the things we discuss might change your life. For others, this approach might not be for you. And that's OK. This isn't a one-size-fits-all problem, so it doesn't have a one-size-fits-all solution. No matter where you are in your relationship to food, I'm here to tell you there *is* a way out of that insanity. Help, healing, and hope are possible—and I want to help you find them.

This book is divided into three parts that address a holistic approach and plan for conquering food issues. In Part I, we'll get into the nitty-gritty of diagnosing food addiction, including the science behind it, the questions it raises, and the various means of support available for those who need it. Part II builds upon the knowledge gleaned in Part I and moves into action steps. This is where you'll learn all about how to pick and craft a food plan—your Satisfied Food Plan—which will keep you on the path of health and healing, based on your lifestyle and needs. Part III provides you with the resources you'll need for your food plan: yummy, healthy recipes that will keep you satisfied and nourished for a lifetime!

Because the journey of conquering food issues involves so many important nutritional considerations, I've collaborated with experienced dietitian Jackie Mack. You'll benefit greatly

INTRODUCTION

from her insights. She also contributed some of her own favorite recipes!

Whether you are a food addict (and if you're unsure what that means, read on!) or are simply looking to cultivate a healthier relationship with food, we've got all the resources in the pages that follow to help you kick harmful food habits to the curb in favor of sustainable, lifelong healthy food practices.

PART One

DIAGNOSE THE PROBLEM

CHAPTER 1

So How Do I Start?

Now that you've seen some new language around the reality of food addiction, I'm sure one question is blaring in your mind: so how do I eat *well*?

I have been working in the overeating recovery/food addiction space for over thirty years now, and the entire time there has been no true consensus about how people should eat once they are in recovery. I like to call it the Big Food Fight. Many people have (understandably) incredibly strong opinions, with a lot of people advocating for a one-size-fits-all method.

I don't believe in a one-size-fits-all model, and I'll even go one step further: I'm actually highly opposed to people imposing that type of thinking onto others, because it's something I had to wrestle through myself. In the first stages of my food recovery, I encountered many people who believed that if you didn't eat in "such and such a way" now that you were in recovery, you weren't in recovery. I bumped up against a lot of hardcore, black-and-white thinking, and it just didn't sit right with me.

My first few years in recovery were difficult. Changing my eating habits was agony after so many years eating to excess, and I definitely struggled, despite my desire to change. It took me two and half years to completely get off sugar and highly processed foods for good, after many, many relapses and slow steps toward change.

MAYBE I JUST HAVE A SWEET TOOTH?

You might be wondering: *Am I a food addict? Or do I just have a sweet tooth?* And now is definitely the right time to ask yourself that! Regardless of where you fall on the spectrum of eating issues—whether you are indeed a food addict, have an unhealthy relationship with food, have a sweet tooth, are prediabetic, etc.—what follows in this book will still be of use to you. Let's take a stab at diagnosing the problem. Ask yourself these questions, and try to answer as honestly as you can:

1. When I eat sugar/white flour/highly processed foods (e.g., cake, cookies, pizza, pasta, etc.), do I feel that I am in control? Am I able to stop once I have consumed the amount I set out to eat?

SO HOW DO I START?

2. Am I able to enjoy sweet treats in moderation—at weddings, on birthdays, etc.? Or does eating treats/sugar never stop at just one treat?
3. When I think about food, what feelings do I experience? Do I feel anxious, out of control, chaotic, overwhelmed? Do I feel in control of my eating, or do I feel like my eating is controlling me?
4. Is eating sugar/white flour/highly processed foods becoming unmanageable?
5. Do I think about the next time I will have treats or fast food all day, every day?

If you answered no to the first two questions and yes to the latter three, you may want to investigate further the possibility that you may have a food addiction. If that results in big feelings, don't worry—you're not alone, and there is so much love and support coming your way in this book, as well as a clear path out of addiction and into freedom. There is hope and help available to you, and I want to be part of that process.

If you answered yes to the first two questions and no to the latter three, and you still picked up this book, you might be looking for help with your relationship with food. Maybe you went to the doctor recently and discovered you were prediabetic. Maybe you feel you have, as one friend likes to call it, "an over-appreciation of chocolate chip cookies." Maybe you just want to get off highly processed foods, and you're looking for a food plan focused on doing so (one you can stick to).

Just like with drugs or alcohol, there are actual food *addicts*, but there are also food *abusers*. It's important to understand the difference between the two. The life of a food *addict* is completely controlled and run by their relationship with food. They are constantly thinking about the next time they will eat donuts or a big greasy pizza, and they can never have "just one cookie" or "just one slice of cake." They obsess about food and might be stuck in a cycle of bingeing, followed by feelings of shame and guilt, possibly followed by some form of purging, followed by more bingeing, and so on. This often results in secretive behavior, lying about what/when they have eaten when asked about it, and intense feelings of isolation, shame, and guilt. The food addict is completely out of control, and food is their drug of choice in trying to find control (like we saw in my own story).

Food *abusers* are a much broader category. They can certainly overindulge in sweet treats, but they are not controlled by them. Let's take my friend Gina, for example. She went to the doctor a few years ago and discovered that she was pre-diabetic. She loves her sweet treats and all kinds of yummy bread, but after getting this diagnosis, she understood she had to make some significant changes to the way that she ate. She decided to follow a Whole30 diet, which worked really well

SO HOW DO I START?

for her. After some trial and error, she found that she was able to still have pizza with her husband every few weeks and eat a slice of cake at weddings and then hop right back on to her Whole30 plan. She's able to stay healthy while still enjoying a treat now and then. She can eat treats in moderation, without the occasional indulgence throwing her whole life into chaos.

When it comes to figuring out whether you're a food *addict* or a food *abuser*, the main question you are seeking to answer is: How firm do my food boundaries need to be? If you're reading this book and you fall into the food abuser category, you likely need to find some firmer boundaries that still offer some flexibility. If you're a food addict, you *do* need firm boundaries, and those boundaries need to stay firm.

Regardless of which camp you find yourself in, the methods and tools Jackie and I offer in this book will help you experience peace in your relationship with food. We are focused on helping you discover the right plan that fits perfectly into your life based on your needs, and we know that with God's help, freedom from any battle with food is possible.

FIRST STEPS

Let me give you a broad outline of how I eventually found my own personal meal plan. It began with me simply trying to stop eating sugar, which, as I said, did not happen overnight (far from it!). This was around the time that people in recovery circles were recommending eating three meals a day with no snacking in between, so that was the next thing I tried: three meals only, no late-night snacking or midday munchies. To be clear, these meals were still unhealthy, too-large portions full of white flour, but they were a step in the right direction. Everything began to come together when a friend in my support group showed me some meal plan options.

This is when I began to learn what normal portions were, because I began weighing and measuring my food. This concept is a great example of something that is too rigid for some people, but at the beginning of my recovery, weighing and measuring served as a useful tool in figuring out how much belonged on my plate and what would be more nourishing food.

These meal plan suggestions cut out sugar and white flour, of course, but they placed a huge emphasis on portion size, as well as the correct ratios of protein, fat, carbs, veggies, et al., on my plate. From the get-go, I found myself failing pretty miserably. The rigidness of having to measure and weigh all of my food seemed almost as crazy-making as the food behaviors I was trying to escape.

Don't get me wrong—learning about appropriate portion sizes and food group ratios *is* important. For most of us entering food addiction recovery, we don't know the first thing about how much to eat of something good, and it's incredibly

SO HOW DO I START?

valuable to take the time to learn about the differences between proteins, starches, fats, and so on, and how best to incorporate them into our meals. I credit this time in my life to my present understanding of what good portion sizes are, and I learned a lot about what to put on my plate. And let me be clear: many people need this much structure in order to stay in recovery. They have found freedom in the structure, and I celebrate and support them.

This is a great time to pause and say: wherever you can start is the right place to start. It took me two and a half *years* to really get my meal plan together. I'm giving you the broad outline of my own experience so you can get a few ideas and examples, but start where you can. If you're a person who can jump into hardcore structure right away, great! We are going to get a bit more into that shortly. But if you have to start slow, then start slow. The important thing is just to start.

For me (and for many other people), this weighing-and-measuring type of constant vigilance over each and every detail of each and every meal didn't work. I went through a lot of trial and error over those first years to get where I am today in my approach. I learned from other people in recovery, and I was game to try all kinds of advice. Every week in my recovery meeting, I listened intently to descriptions of the food plans others were incorporating, and I'd show up the following week to see how it was playing out in their lives. Some approaches were too messy, some too constricting. Some things I tried felt akin to a diet without enough calories, which I knew for me personally was a slippery slope right back into bingeing and purging.

But no matter which combination I tried, I always found myself bristling against the idea that abstinence in food recovery had to be rigid. I knew there had to be a way to lean into the abundant life God wants for us, a way to truly enjoy food that was good for me, all while no longer stuffing myself to the gills with greasy pizza and gallons of ice cream.

Which brings me to the whole point of this book in your hands: I knew that I needed my meals to feel *satisfying*. For me, a life where I was chained to a hard-and-fast set of rules was just another type of bondage like the thing I was fleeing. My dips and forays into all the different food plans I tried led me to my Satisfied Food Plan recovery philosophy, which I hope and pray can bring joy and freedom to your life. Taking the long road to get to this realization was ultimately beneficial, as I learned what my needs are calorically and nutritionally. And I think the same is possible for you!

YOUR UNIQUE FOOD PLAN

As you may be understanding by this point, my food plan philosophy is that *you* will be one of the authors of your specific

SO HOW DO I START?

food plan—because you are a unique person with unique needs. You'll craft it with the help, support, and guidance of people who have gone before you, because we all need help. Some trial and error will be required. Lots of it! But I hope to mitigate that somewhat, early in your food addiction recovery process, by explaining some of your options and the many support resources you can use.

I can't stress this enough: join a support group as soon as you can. This is really the place your food plan gets started. It's also great to seek advice and guidance from a nutritionist who understands food addiction, and often you can find one through the network of your support group.

I know how overwhelming this seems. Take a deep breath. If strictness around food makes you feel shame, find a nutritionist who has a relaxed approach. If you need a lot of structure, seek out someone in your support group who has shared something about that in their own journey. Embrace being teachable; embrace your need for help. Your addiction can't be the guide here.

One of the first steps in the right direction is to think about and identify your specific trigger foods. Take a minute and ask yourself, *What foods do I struggle with? Are they foods that are salty, sweet, fatty, crunchy, chewy? Or is it more the quantity of food rather than particular foods?*

THE SATISFIED GUIDE TO EATING WELL

Write down a few foods you currently have trouble with or had trouble with in the past.

_____

_____

_____

_____

PLUG AND PLAY

My philosophy about food eating plans is ultimately a plug-and-play method: if you have the right amounts of protein, veggies, fats, and starches on your plate, you can fill it with an infinite amount of delicious possibilities and combinations.

So, what is the right portion of each of those food groups? Even this will look different for each of us! In the resources I've already mentioned, you can find the appropriate balance for each of your meals. It's important to listen to sound advice from people you trust and figure out what works for you.*

---

* There are plenty of authors whose work you can turn to as you begin to approach food addiction. Dr. Robert H. Lustig, Dr. Nicole Avena, Dr. Mark Hyman, Dr. David Wiss, and Dr. Gabor Maté are all great resources. In your area you can also find many free resources and groups, such as Overeaters Anonymous (www.oa.org/find-a-meeting).

SO HOW DO I START?

Some of you might already be discouraged by the prospect of a plate full of vegetables. I get it! I was raised in a house where the only vegetables we ate came in cans. I grew up *hating* vegetables. Who wanted that yucky, salty stuff when you could have cake and ice cream and cookies? I had no idea how delicious broccoli, green beans, or sweet potatoes could taste until I began my food recovery journey. Believe me: vegetables can taste delicious! There are all kinds of ways to prepare them (feel free to peek ahead at the recipe section if you need a little bit of encouragement). Again, we are taking this one step at a time. It's a *process*.

With some honest inventory, a bit of bravery, an abundance of God's help, and the encouragement of people who have gone before you, I know you can craft the perfect meal plan for your recovery journey. Over the years, I have learned how to look at my food and figure out what portions are best for me personally. I've also learned how to prepare veggies and proteins in some truly delicious ways. Inside this plug-and-play method, there's so much freedom. A huge weight was lifted off my shoulders after I took the time to get to know the point of the food on my plate and understand my relationship to it. Food is meant to nourish us—not drive us crazy. I have a problem overeating *sugar*; I don't have a problem overeating stir-fry. Believe me, you can learn how to trust yourself, too, after you admit the reality of your problem and need for help. It may sound daunting at the outset, but it's so, so worth it.

PICK WHAT STICKS

For me, a food plan is all about *routine*. Creating a routine you can stick to, under the lens of a plug-and-play method that works specifically for you, means you can go into every week knowing exactly what you need to plan for your meals. And doing so will give you confidence to face any life situation and know the best option for you.

All of my meals have the same amount of fruits, veggies, starches, proteins, and fats, with very little variation. The food itself varies, of course, but the proportion and ratios do not. After so many years of practice, I have a little mental picture of what my plate should look like at mealtime, which means even when I travel or go to a restaurant, I can figure out exactly what I need based on that picture. It's such a gift of flexibility, because while there's an "exact" frame of reference I'm using, I don't have to *meet* it exactly every time. I've done the groundwork of knowing what the right foods and portions are, which means I can plug them into any situation and find something that works.

I don't know about you, but routine empowers me. If I don't have to think about my food, it keeps me out of trouble. It's so incredibly freeing to have food in its right place; it's the exact opposite of the obsessive thoughts that plagued me during my entire youth. As far as I'm concerned, boundaries and routine are sanity keepers. They prohibit me from eating haphazardly or emotionally, and they empower me to advocate for myself in all kinds of situations.

Here are some examples of my personal Satisfied Food Plan, ones I've learned through the School of Falling on My Face over the years. . . .

I know that I can't sleep in, because that will throw off my meal balance. If I throw off the timing of my meals during the day, that will throw off my appetite. I have to eat the same portions, and I should aim to eat at close to the same time every day, because if I overeat or undereat, that could set me off. If it's not my mealtime, I don't haphazardly snack or graze. The only time I eat is during the times I have planned out for my meals—that's it.

Every week, I do a lot of well-thought-out meal prep. Is it rigid? No! It's coming from a place of knowledge. This is another part of the process that took me a long time to figure out. I'll be honest: it's still not my favorite part of recovery. But I have learned from others how to make it more enjoyable. I call a friend or I play worship music as a I chop and mix my meals for the week. And now, I don't mind it as much, because I love having healthy food all ready to go. It's worth the effort.

Yes, at first it involves planning and dedicated time set aside. But eventually it becomes habit.

For me now, going into my day without a food plan is a trigger for confusion. It's a setup for one of my old spirals: "What am I gonna do about food?" I need quiet in my head where food is concerned. I've found so, so much peace in my meal prep practice.

If that means packing my lunch the night before, then I do it. I don't want to be figuring out something on the fly because of a lack of preparedness. You truly can't *over*prepare.

Have I made mistakes over the years? Of course! But I always have a Plan B. For example, I used to keep a jar of almond butter and some rice cakes in my office closet in case I forgot my lunch. The last thing I wanted to do on a thirty-minute lunch break was have to eat fast food. And we *don't* have to eat fast food. We can learn the location of nearby restaurants where we can buy a takeout salad or other options that work with our food plan.

Remember: this is an addiction. You have to treat it that seriously; the risk is simply too high for relapse if you don't give it the attention and care it requires.

I go to great lengths to protect my food plan and habits—I have to. My recovery requires it. I never, ever want to suffer that insanity again, and I now know for sure what will trigger that confusion for me personally.

SO HOW DO I START?

Another huge need for me is always having a fully stocked fridge. I'd rather have "extra" of the good stuff than be in a situation where I can't make dinner because I don't have vegetables on hand. I don't operate well when I don't have what I need. And there's no shame in that. For me, having my food in its right place is like having water, electricity, or any other life necessity. It's a "must," not some option to play with.

As I have learned through working with clients and groups for the past thirty years, this is crucial: you must understand how necessary preparedness is to your recovery—understand what trips your wires so you don't get caught up in what could be an incredibly easy fix with the right prep. I can't count how many clients I've treated who have come into my office thinking they don't need a food plan, that they can wing it through willpower, only to find themselves relapsing.

One client in particular comes to mind. She had "successfully" completed a new diet she was trying, and it had run its course right around Thanksgiving. As she followed this diet, she lost roughly a hundred pounds and felt that she would be able to enjoy sugar again in moderation now that she'd had a reset. At her family's gathering, she cut herself a tiny sliver of pie at the end of her meal. This client came into my office a few days later, thrilled that she'd been able to pull it off—"just one piece!" Unfortunately, she found herself on a slippery slope from Thanksgiving into Christmas: she started playing a bit more loosely with her food and indulging more and more—at parties, at family gatherings, and in other settings. From there, the brakes were off, and before she knew it, she had gained back the hundred pounds and then some.

I share this story not because of the weight loss and gain, but to caution you to consider how little room there is to play with addiction. All of us want to be able to do this on our own willpower, but we've got to learn we simply can't. An alcoholic doesn't take a drink on New Year's Eve just because it's a holiday. Think of it like this: your meal plan is your self-protection from easy dips back into addiction. I know that with certain foods and certain food behaviors, I must protect myself if I want to enjoy a lifetime of success, peace, and freedom in my relationship with food.

YOU CAN ALWAYS FIND AN ALTERNATIVE

You might be thinking, *OK, Dr. Rhona, that's all well and good when I'm prepping my meals for myself and cooking at home, but what do I do when something unexpected comes up? Life happens!* Totally understandable question. Here's another example from my own life: I had to take a blood test for some routine lab work, and I was told I had to drink a super sugary drink in advance of the test. I told them that wouldn't work for me—no overly long explanation needed, just a statement of my

SO HOW DO I START?

needs—and they came up with an alternative. (Don't worry—we'll look into vacations and catered affairs in chapter 9!)

Hear me when I say: you can *always* find an alternative. But you have to ask questions and advocate for yourself. Don't be afraid to ask! Sure, you might feel embarrassed or awkward, or even like you're imposing, but that's simply not the case. If you've spent years and years neglecting your health and needs because of your food addiction, a bit of overcorrection might feel incredibly unnatural. It's all part of the process. Remember, you are in *recovery* for an *addiction*. Don't throw your entire recovery away over a little extra work.

You're not simply on a diet or hoping to lose some weight; you're looking for work-arounds because you don't want to reignite your addiction. Go the extra mile: ask for what you need, and trust that there is always a way through. You are allowed to ask; in fact, your recovery depends on it.

I empathize with how over-the-top this all might sound right now. It's a learning curve for sure, and like all good things, it takes time to find the right rhythm. Lots of it. But I want to encourage you and let you know that for me, all these rhythms and food-prep routines and food behaviors have become as simple and rote as brushing my teeth now. The hardest part is figuring out where to start and how to continue successfully. You're in the right place, and you're not doing this alone.

This process is not just about food. There's almost always a myriad of emotional and spiritual issues attached to any addiction. If you don't face them head-on, you won't understand why you want to eat and what triggers you to do so in an unhealthy way. That's why I wrote this book, and why I have fought so hard for so many years for people to understand that in order to get freedom from food addiction, you have to approach it from a mind-body-spirit perspective. If you are able to view food addiction as something affected by all three of these aspects, and if you're able to get them in balance with one another, you have a chance of sustainable peace in your life that you're never going to find if you just go on another diet.

CHOOSING ABUNDANCE

As you know, my food recovery journey began in a support group. I've detailed for you a bit of how I started approaching my food plan, but I haven't said much about how exactly the purging ultimately stopped for me. One day, during a support group meeting, I shared that I had fallen off the wagon the night before, despite my best efforts to stick to my food plan, and I had ended up bingeing and then starving myself to compensate. Later, when the meeting was over, someone in my circle of support sought me out and suggested that I never overcompensate for my guilt. This was an absolute revelation for me, and it taught me an important lesson: no matter what happened—no matter if I "failed" at my food plan and ending up bingeing, or if I felt completely overwhelmed by all the work ahead of me and longed for a box of donuts—I could always wake up the next day and try again. In other words, if I did end up bingeing, all I had to do was try my food plan again instead of starving myself. She provided me with a pivotal truth for any addict in recovery: we can always pursue replacing old patterns with new patterns, even when we fail.

I fell off the wagon more than once as I pursued recovery—actually, hundreds of times! There were times I felt like I had no idea what I was doing, and the confusion triggered a bingeing and purging spiral, which in turn sent me into a shame spiral and made me doubt I could ever truly recover. But that isn't true. The revelation I've just shared in this story helped me to eliminate compensatory behavior and take responsibility for my recovery in a way that up until that point I simply couldn't.

I also want to encourage you by letting you know that I really, really like what I eat in my life of freedom, and I don't feel deprived. Over time, I've grown to appreciate so many abundant, wonderful foods and recipes and healthy ways of eating that I never would have found otherwise. I love being able to take care of my body through what I eat—not in regard to weight, but through a lens of pursuing health and learning to take care of my body instead of abusing it by cramming it full of unhealthy foods and toxic chemicals. Like anything in life, it's a choice. And I'm choosing abundance. There are truly countless healthy, delicious choices. It has been so redemptive for me learning to expand my palate and finding out just how many great foods are out there. I hadn't known about them because there wasn't room in my appetite or brain for something that wasn't completely destructive.

Here, on the other side of choosing to start, I am able to find something to eat pretty much anywhere that I genuinely like—something that doesn't trip my insanity wire—even when it's not "exactly on my plan." And I fully, wholeheartedly believe the same is true for you. All it takes is that first step—abundance awaits you.

CHAPTER 2

Sugar Addiction

As you have probably noticed by now, this book is based on the premise that for some people, sugar and processed carbohydrates (e.g., white flour, highly processed foods) are scientifically proven to be addictive (just like alcohol, narcotics, etc.).[1] It's crucial to understand this as we make commitments and take first steps toward recovery. The reason what we're doing in this book works is because the whole purpose is to get us out of the endless loop of diets and the various triggering situations we put ourselves in when we don't understand and have a healthy respect for the root cause of the issue. The process of recovering from an addiction is not going on another diet or trying a new health fad. If you are addicted to heroin, you have to completely remove heroin from your life, and eventually, with God's help and your commitment, the heroin cravings go away.

There's plenty of science to back up the idea that sugar can be as addictive as narcotics and alcohol for some people.[2] We're going to take a look at a small sector of it to help deepen your understanding of what exactly is going on in your body and brain in the addictive process.

Let's consider what happens inside your brain when you eat sugar. The pleasure centers light up—they are excited simply by seeing a sugary treat. For someone with an addictive tendency, your brain is significantly more excited[3] than a "normal" person's. For whatever reason, sugar and refined carbohydrates "light up" the addictive brain at an alarmingly higher rate. That might feel unfair, and it's OK to wrestle with that feeling. But it's important to understand this as an impartial fact. We need to understand this information in order to best know how to move forward.

Let's look at a bit more of the science behind the brain of an addictive person. There's a hormone in everyone's brain called *leptin*, which lets you know when you're full. If you have been overeating (bingeing and purging, using crash diets, etc.) for years and years, your brain doesn't have the same cues for satiety as someone who does not abuse food, because you have trained it to tell you you're "full" only after eating way too much food.[4] You have trained your body to accommodate your addiction through years of extending the limit of how much is enough. Take a second to sit with that: addiction affects you at a hormonal level. Talk about all-consuming!

Similarly, another hormone in your brain is *dopamine*, often referred to as the "happy hormone" because it communicates pleasure. Dopamine secretes throughout the body for a variety of reasons, often when we are doing something that delights us—which, for many of us, is the act of eating sugar. Much like leptin, your dopamine regulation can be completely hijacked by the addiction process.[5] When you have extended the amount of sweet things you put into your body over time, it requires more and more of those sweet things to tell your body that you "feel good"—meaning you have trained your body to "need more sweets" in order to get that same dopamine release. Therefore, the pleasure center in your brain has a totally unhealthy rhythm: you continue to need more and more because you have overeaten past the typical limits of what constitutes "feeling good."

REWRITING THE PATHWAYS

So what does this mean for you? With a background of first understanding the science behind addiction, it's just as important to understand how this science informs what triggers you and how it relates to you personally. In order to make a food plan that will keep you strong in recovery, you first need to rewrite these pathways in your brain. You've got to begin at the hormonal level. The easiest way to start is with a clean slate and then to discern for yourself what triggers you and what you can keep in your diet. It's not unlike an elimination diet, where you remove everything that could potentially trip you up and then slowly reintroduce certain foods that could potentially remain in your food plan.

Everyone's sensitivities are different, and as I said in the last chapter, it will take a lot of trial and error to figure out what trips you up the most. For example, some people might be OK with certain alternative flour products and healthy whole grains. For others, those are impossible to manage. You've got to figure out what your limits are, and once you do, you'll better understand why it's so important to respect them.

It may not come as a surprise that this line of thinking is quite controversial in the addiction field. Most people in the food addiction recovery space come from the school of thought that I mentioned in the last chapter: *rigidly remove from your diet everything that could potentially be triggering, no exceptions; otherwise, you cannot say you are in recovery.*

While I deeply respect my colleagues and understand where they're coming from, I do differ from them here. For example, lots of people think you have to cut out flour completely—there's not opportunity for trial and error. Yet I can comfortably eat healthy flour products made with whole ingredients while many of my clients are not able to do the same.

There is a continuum of sensitivity for all of us, which makes things complicated. That's why it's tempting to just cut out everything. If you want to play it as safe as possible, I encourage you not to play with anything that might overcomplicate your food recovery. That is absolutely in line with my philosophy, because it comes from a place of self-knowledge. You have to do what *you* figure out is best for you. That's why I encourage trial and error.

For example, if you know flour isn't an issue for you, then you may be able to try out some of the healthy, 100-percent whole grain, no-sugar options—or better yet, try sprouted grains. An abundance of delicious foods falls into these categories, and they can be a delightful addition to your food plan if they're not a problem for you. What's more, they can help create excitement around crafting your food plan because of the variety they bring. They can help heal your relationship with food and remind you of the many ways God designed food to nourish us.

(On that note, some of you may be wondering about food labels in general and how they inform our ability to nourish ourselves. Fear not, we will get to that in a later chapter. We'll also learn what it means when we say a food is "processed" and how to differentiate it from what isn't.)

If any kind of detox sounds overwhelming to you at this point, don't worry, and don't lose faith! We'll have plenty of options of how to get started in Part II.

For now, the goal of explaining all this is to help you get rid of whatever will keep you in your cravings, and therefore in bondage. Reducing cravings is the first, most crucial part of this food addiction recovery battle. The sooner you clearly understand what triggers you and what doesn't, the sooner you'll be able to meaningfully craft a food plan you can sustain. This isn't necessarily about weight loss, although switching out junk food for vegetables will of course have some physical outcomes.

As I hope you are beginning to understand, sugar is highly addictive. White flour is highly addictive. Highly processed food is highly addictive. Which brings me to our next point of contention that you will have to experiment with yourself: artificial sweeteners. This is one of the hot topics that keeps food professionals in the Big Food Fight. Many believe sweeteners are too much like "the real thing" and therefore shouldn't be trifled with; ergo some professionals and recovery groups have a big fat *no!* for them. Others contend that a limited, scheduled amount of stevia (or monk fruit or other natural options) might be OK and help keep people "in" the process.

This is part of what we're figuring out here in this book: does a little stevia in your coffee help your recovery, or does it simply create a craving for something sweeter, and send you off the deep end?

As you can see, there's a lot of minutiae to wade through to figure out what will and won't work for you. My suggestion is to start with a month of completely clearing out everything that could even remotely be considered a trigger—mints, gums, artificial sweeteners—and detox from anything and everything. Along the way, pay attention to what comes up in you. Maybe keep a journal of what you find yourself missing or obsessing over. Pay attention to what your body is trying to tell you, keeping in mind that it's in a correction process.

After the month is up, evaluate where you are and check in with yourself. Review what you've journaled, take stock of what you think you can safely bring back in—and make a plan for what you can't. For instance, if you know that mints are ultimately going to be a problem for you, switch out eating mints for brushing your teeth or using mouthwash in the middle of the day. Think of this month as a reset and a detox to truly clean out your system from *anything* that could be triggering and keeping you in addiction. This is your best bet for accurately evaluating what will and will not keep you in the addictive process. Again, I know it may sound daunting at the onset, but I promise you, progress is possible! And I promise good things—life-saving things—are waiting on the other side.

Remember, the brain chemistry of a person with addictive tendencies is different from the brain of someone without them. Addicted brains are habituated so that "just one treat" will always lead to an excessive amount. When we do the work of training our brain to go in a different direction, we begin to give our brain a new pathway. How cool is that? You can train your brain, with perseverance, to crave what is ultimately good for you. As a result, you will learn to love your new way, and you will find satisfaction and happiness in your new pathway out of the addiction process.

Simply put, you can't be in both worlds; once the door to addiction is closed, it needs to stay closed. Again, it's important for you to understand that your addiction exists on a cellular, brain-specific level. You need to change your brain for good and teach it how to live healthy and well, not overcome by addiction. We have lived in a world always looking for that next fix in the form of a candy bar or a pint of ice cream. But with a mind-body-spirit mindset, we are going to learn so many new ways of dealing with our food—and therefore our lives—that will keep us balanced and healthy.

EVERY DAY IS A CHANCE TO START AGAIN

I hope this helps you understand a bit better why I suggest total abstinence from anything and everything for at least a month. We need a break from this toxic way of living so we can have a chance to regulate and heal. The body is so beautifully adaptable, but it takes time and concentrated effort. We need to take care of ourselves to make up for so many years of abusing our bodies. If we don't, we will only continue to flood our brain with warped signals from chemicals and hormones designed by God to give us good things and regulate our bodies into flourishing. Thankfully, He made our bodies capable of healing, and there *is* hope. We can teach our brains new things, and we *can* teach our bodies hormonal balance using healthy and whole foods.

If you're feeling discouraged, you're not alone. Even though I was truly desperate when I came into recovery, a part of me was terrified I would never enjoy healthy food as I began the process of changing the way I ate. Even though I *knew* my addiction was ruining my life, I was in many ways afraid I would never truly be able to give up the only foods I had been eating for years and replace them with yucky healthy food. I'm so glad I stuck it out. It is totally possible to experience enjoyment with healthy food. And, if you can believe it, you *don't* need decadent food in high doses in order to enjoy eating. You will be amazed at what can be recovered—but you have to trust me to go through this process with full commitment.

Like any addiction, the detox portion can be difficult. Remember: you're training your body for a whole new way of living. Have some grace with yourself! If you fall off the wagon, that doesn't mean you're a hopeless case. There is no need to overcompensate for feeling guilty. Each day is an opportunity to start again. I promise you; it just takes some time. What feels impossible now will get easier, and so many people who felt the same way you may be feeling now have made it to the other side.

EVERYONE IS DIFFERENT, BUT ADDICTION IS THE SAME

The purpose of this book is to heal our brains—to stop the cravings, address addictions, and get us to a place where we can have real, lasting freedom. I will stress this the entire book, but it bears repeating: everyone is different. Some of you will only need a few days of abstinence from sugar and highly processed foods to feel the cravings flee; for others it could take years. The science suggests that the average amount of time it takes for a craving to disappear in an abstinence mentality is about two months, or sixty-six days.[6] The main thing to understand is the need for totality in abstinence. As in, even a little bit of sugar is too much. Remember, this is an addiction just like any other addiction. One drink for an alcoholic is enough to reignite the addictive process, and it's the same with the addiction we're dealing with here.

Remember the story from the last chapter about my client who had the tiny piece of pie at Thanksgiving, and that was all it took to send her right back off the deep end? It's never just "one little treat" for food addicts. There are, of course, people who can successfully eat sugar in moderation, just as there are people who can successfully drink alcohol in moderation without being addicted. But chances are, if you are reading this book, you are not one of those people. It's never just one piece of pie for us; it's the whole pie, over and over again, every time we try to deny the fact that this is a place in our lives where we are out of control.

CHAPTER 3

Approaching Your Food Plan—It's All About Mindset

Perhaps the most difficult part of starting the food addiction recovery process is adjusting your mindset. As we discussed in the last chapter, the pathways in our brain have been habituated into certain routes and behaviors. It goes hand in hand that our mindset has also been conditioned by our lifetime of behaviors and beliefs. In this case, I'm talking about the internalized messaging that any change in your diet intake should be focused on weight loss. This point of focus has to be readjusted. You want to shift your internal messaging toward what your food plan is ultimately about: ending cravings and addictive eating patterns and habits.

This is a huge (and hard!) shift for most people. We all have a lifetime of experiences and longings that inform how we arrive at this mindset. In addition, the world is constantly telling us to lose weight. And most of us who are addicted to food *want* to lose weight. Which, to be clear, is not a bad goal in itself if you are looking to become healthier. It just can't be the motivating force behind your recovery, because if things don't go your way as fast as you want them to, you'll find yourself right back in the addictive pattern.

We have a lot of messaging from diet culture in our heads to sift through. Many of us have tried all kinds of fad diets over the years in our exhausting quest to conquer food. In our dieting, we've learned all about how carbs and fats are bad, how we shouldn't be eating too many calories, how such and such food is a miracle fat burner . . . .

The information and opinions are endless, and incredibly confusing. And they are particularly damaging to people like us who already have our own twisted thinking about food, especially if we're anxious about losing weight.

Let's be honest here. From the outset, we all still want that magic cure for losing weight, whatever trick or behavior we have convinced ourselves will do it for us (no carbs, liquid fasts, intermittent fasting—again, the options are endless). If any of these diets were really going to work in a sustainable way, you wouldn't be reading (and I wouldn't be writing) this book.

APPROACHING YOUR FOOD PLAN—IT'S ALL ABOUT MINDSET

For so many of us, we've managed to succeed at the various programs we've tried . . . until we haven't. These programs and promises change every generation, and every new promise is always backed by scientists and doctors. But if that's the case, why does the diagnosis keep changing?

It's important to look at the messaging we receive and take stock of our own reality in the midst of it. Sure, it's likely that you have successfully lost weight when trying a handful of programs over the years, but I'm guessing there's been no sustainability. These diets are designed to be quick fixes to get us drastic results (not unlike hits of dopamine in our brain with something sweet). This lack of sustainability is why food addiction tends to win out: Life interrupts after our thirty-day juice fasts. A holiday arrives during a maintenance period. A celebration at work involves cake and ice cream.

We don't realize that the food we've been avoiding is not just "something that could make us fat"—it's addictive.

Your defenses are especially low if you've been depriving yourself for a long time, which makes it that much easier for the addictive process to reignite over something that might appear small or intended to be a brief indulgence after hard work.

I can't tell you how many clients in my office over the years have tried a diet, gone to a birthday party at the end of the dieting period, enjoyed a small slice of cake, and then gained back every pound they'd lost (and then some). Everyone thinks they are the exception, even after learning for themselves that's not the case. As food addicts, it's all or nothing. When we reintroduce any piece of food that's sugary, processed, or full of white flour, we fall right back into the addiction pattern.

Remember the pleasure centers in your brain. The second our brain gets the signal that it's tasting sugar, it goes bonkers and the cravings are completely reactivated. Whatever work was accomplished on your diet disappears the second a treat is in your mouth. The step between "just one bite" and absolutely losing control is extremely short.

Just because your friend can complete a round of Whole30 and then reintegrate certain food groups back into their diet doesn't mean you can do the same if you have addictive tendencies. Again, if you're an addict you can't do moderation of addictive foods. I know it may seem like I'm overemphasizing this, but it's so important to understand if you want to have lasting change. You've got years of diet culture in your head that you're working against, giving you endless mixed messages about what you can and can't eat and what you can and can't do with your food. What's more, we also live in a culture saturated with messaging about "treating yourself," often with food, which is crazy-making in tandem with the diet culture. But if you're a food addict, none of that messaging matters. And clearly, none of it is working.

APPROACHING YOUR FOOD PLAN—IT'S ALL ABOUT MINDSET

So, if you wholeheartedly pursue recovery and a Satisfied Food Plan, will you lose weight? More than likely. It doesn't take a doctor to know that if you swap out greasy pizza and cookies with healthy proteins and vegetables, the change affects what you look like. But that's just a side effect, not the *point* of changing your behavior. And if it *is* the focus of your pursuit, it just becomes another diet in the arsenal you've already tried, leading to the same result. It simply won't work. The mindset has to change. We are looking at and pursuing a true, lasting lifestyle shift—a way to end cravings and compulsive eating for good so we can live lives free of insanity. It's important to understand that when we build a food plan, the focus is different from anything we've done before.

BE HONEST WITH YOURSELF

Another part of the mindset shift is radical self-honesty. You've got to get real about what trips you up, and commit to doing whatever it takes to remove these hindrances (with plenty of grace along the way). If you know a certain food has kept you in the struggle (your "gateway drug," if you will, back into the addictive process), you'll need to address that tendency in your food plan. I can't stress this enough: moderation isn't going to cut it in the recovery process. If I eat a cookie "in moderation," that cookie is calling my name all day long. If I don't eat cookies, they don't call me.

We need to directly address the food-related messages our brain is sending. That way we can to rewire it to understand what food is intended to bring into our bodies—nourishment, vitality, energy—so we are not constantly fixating on the next time we can eat and what we'll eat once we get there. We have to address our relationship and connection to food itself. When we do so, we may end up noticing some habits and patterns that we didn't realize were part of the problem.*

For some people, simply replacing junk food with healthy food doesn't necessarily work if the bad habit stays the same. One example of this is all-day snacking or grazing. Even if you're snacking all day long on celery and hummus instead of potato chips or candy, you're not really addressing the habit itself: disordered eating. We can't be playing with food throughout the day if we're looking to quiet the noise in our heads. We need to make sure that our meals are truly satisfying, and that we don't eat food we don't absolutely love as some kind of recompense. If we simply swap addictive foods with food we "think of" as healthy, it's going to feel like a diet where we're

---

* Dr. Mark Hyman is a great resource on this topic. He has a wealth of materials available on his website, www.drhyman.com.

constantly looking for replacements. Instead, we're in pursuit of something sustainable.

You want to eat your dinner knowing that it was delicious, that you really liked it, that it was satisfying and good for you. You want to look forward to meals without abusing food. It's a totally different mentality when you fully embrace it. The idea of eating well and being satisfied, of leaning into abundance instead of simply looking for quick fixes and shortcuts, totally changes the game.

ADDRESSING YOUR FULLNESS NEEDS

I'll say it again: the point of the food plan you will craft is to establish healthy boundaries with food and shut down addictive and emotional eating. We are learning how to plan what we eat and when we will eat it, and to stick with the plan we know works for us. We want to plan what we eat, and eat what we plan—and that's it. If that's the case, then we definitely need to make sure we are getting what we need in our plan so we can stick to it successfully for a lifetime of freedom and peace.

A huge part of crafting your food plan effectively will involve addressing what your fullness needs are. This can be especially difficult in light of all the ideas we are working against, because we've been taught for so long that to be thin is to be hungry. Again, we are not looking for weight loss as our goal. Release that from your thinking. You want to be full and nourished by foods you enjoy and look forward to! That way, you don't kick-start the chaotic ideation around food and eating when you realize, "Oh, I didn't have enough at lunch. I need to add more food in." If you address your fullness needs at the start, you're setting yourself up not to have to figure it out on the go, thus mitigating the risk of dipping back into the addictive process.

On a related note, if you are crafting a meal plan that doesn't include snacks because you know that's a trigger for a poor eating habit, then you need to make sure lunch has everything you need. Again, it's all a process, and you might not innately know your satiety level after so many years of abusing it. But I'll say it again: *you've got this*. Take your time figuring this out, and your efforts will have lasting effects. We are training ourselves to calm the obsessive loops that exist in our heads and live with good food boundaries, only eating what we know will boost our health and not trigger addictiveness.

MAKING EVERY MEAL COUNT

This is where the serious trial and error comes in. It might take you a year to really begin to figure out what healthy foods you like and the best ways for you to prepare them. Figuring

APPROACHING YOUR FOOD PLAN—IT'S ALL ABOUT MINDSET

out portions can be similarly tricky, especially when the goal behind eating them is being satisfied, not losing weight. Take heart in that the foods we are learning to love and enjoy are not addictive the way sugar is. Sugar (in the additive form) and processed foods are man-made, but whole foods were designed by God to nourish and satisfy us. This boundary of not eating processed foods means that our temptations are held at bay.

I should note here: another important area to pay attention to during your trial and error is fruit. Fruit should absolutely be part of your meal plan. However, as you cultivate your new mindset, you don't want fruit to hijack your food plan with sweetness. There are people for whom some fruits (like grapes or dried fruit) can be a trigger, and they also can affect some people's appetite.

Again, everything comes down to self-knowledge and self-honesty. You have to get real about what triggers you, and you have to get curious and brave about learning the rhythms of your body: your satiety levels, your glycemic responses,* and much more. All these contribute to your ultimate goal: satisfaction without triggering cravings.

---

* Again, Dr. Mark Hyman is a great resource for this, as are Dr. Robert Lustwig and Dr. David Wiss.

Quick Tips w/ Dr. Rhona: Why Should I Eat Real Food?

- As Dr. Mark Hyman is known to say, food is medicine. Eating real food vastly improves your health throughout your whole body![7]
- Processed food has often been stripped of the nutrients that exist in real, raw foods (not to mention mixing in all kinds of man-made chemicals and additives). Eating real food means you are getting the most possible nutrition and keeping additives and chemicals out of your body.
- Your body was designed to digest real foods that occur naturally. That means when you eat real food, your body actually knows what to do with it and can break it down in the healthiest, most beneficial way.
- Quality beats quantity every time. It's not about *how* much you eat, but *what* you are eating.
- Processed food fills you up in quick spurts followed by energy crashes and cravings, but real foods keep you full and satisfied between meals. We're all about that!

APPROACHING YOUR FOOD PLAN—IT'S ALL ABOUT MINDSET

When addiction abates, consequently so will weight, but I encourage you to stay off the scale at first as you craft and begin to experiment with your food plan. Again, it's just not the point. And frankly, it can be discouraging if you don't see what you "expected" right away. In addition, weight is not necessarily a good indicator of what's going on in your body. Give yourself the freedom and space to arrive at a place that works for you.

The intention of this chapter *is* intention—shutting down addiction, getting our heads right, and shifting the focus off weight and onto solutions that last and support our lifelong flourishing. It's a seismic shift! Some of us have never, ever thought of food or our bodies this way. It takes dedicated effort if you have lived your life in weight obsession. But how many of us have ever made real change (internal or external) using ineffective thinking? How many of us have tried the latest craze in a desperate attempt to make ourselves thinner, only to end up right back where we started? As you know from reading my story, it never worked for me. And that's why I'm here and want so badly for you to join me.

Take the focus off weight loss and put it on simply eating well. I promise you: your life can truly change.

CHAPTER 4

Emotional Eating

Before we delve into all the ins and outs of your food plan and longer recovery journey, I want to address what is likely an issue for anyone who comes across this book: emotional eating. This concept affects almost everyone, but it affects us food addicts more deeply than most.

We are not going to do a deep dive into this topic in this book, as I go in-depth in some of my other books, including *Satisfied*[8] and *The Satisfied Workbook*.[9] If, after this chapter, you still have questions or areas of confusion, or you simply want to learn more about handling your emotional eating, I would encourage you to check them out. There's so much in these books about the emotional aspects of recovery. I hope they, too, can help you on your recovery journey, no matter where you are on it.

WHAT DO I DO WHEN "LIFE HAPPENS"?

As a therapist, I often see people who have taken significant strides toward recovery—and then life happens. They've been putting in the effort, working their program, sometimes even starting and implementing their food plans, and then some unforeseen situation sends them off the rails. Maybe it's something major and life-changing like a breakup, a difficult time for their child, a job loss, or a death in the family. Sometimes it's more minor, like a disagreement with their spouse or run-of-the-mill stress at work. Challenges run the gamut; we all know life provides no shortage of emotional interruptions. And because we as food addicts have spent so many years and developed so many patterns of looking to food to solve our problems, these emotional interruptions often slip us up and slow our recovery. We look to food as an old familiar release from feelings and situations we would rather not face.

Something small and simple might occur, and you find yourself in the cupboard raiding your child's school-lunch snack bags or rushing to the grocery store for a half gallon of ice cream. You hear yourself saying, "I couldn't help it—I had to eat!" despite all the hard work you've put in. It's so easy to do and so understandable. Sometimes we'll do anything to shut down our emotions and get out of the situation. Even if we've put in some good work, our automatic response takes over, and we eat.

As the name suggests, these responses are *emotional*. Once again, most of us have spent our whole lives using food to stuff our emotions down rather than deal with them. It's important to keep in mind that giving in to an episode of emotional eating does *not* mean you have thrown your recovery out the window. I'm living proof; I fell on my face so many times when I first started my recovery, I can't even count them! It took me a full three years to completely commit to my life change, and combating emotional eating was one of the biggest obstacles along the way. Ultimately, I learned to look to three anchors when those life interruptions came: my relationship with God, a support system that worked for me, and my food plan. And I know for a fact that when these three things are in order in your own life, your recovery will become your new habit.

YOUR ANCHORS

The first anchor—your relationship with God—is the most personal of the three, and the one I'll spend the least time on here and in the next chapter (again, I go more deeply into this spiritual aspect of recovery in other books). As with everything in the recovery process, there are no shortcuts here. Leaning on God in this vulnerable time is the only path to freedom and peace. If you're not plugged into your faith community, I encourage you to find ways to become involved. Make sure you are meditating on God's Word daily and bringing everything to Him in prayer. No offering is too small. He cares deeply about who you are and what goes on in your life. Even if you feel like you are praying the same prayers over and over again, keep at it. He is your constant companion and support. You can't do this on your own, and blessedly, you don't have to.

Similarly, a good support network is crucial. We'll get into this in later chapters, but as a reminder: you can't do recovery alone! You've got to surround yourself with people who understand what you're going through, who have walked the path and are a little further ahead of you and can encourage you. Get plugged into a support group where you can share your experiences of emotional eating and be met with people who can advise and support you. The more you're around people who have gone through these same experiences, the more you'll truly understand that recovery is possible, and that no matter how you're feeling that day, you are not alone. The power of example can't be overstated.[*] I never would have

---

[*] Brené Brown, the revered shame researcher, author, and speaker, has a wonderful article about the positive and negative effects the people you have in your life can have on your sobriety and her own experience finding supports that worked for her in her sobriety journey: "What Being Sober Has Meant to Me," at www.brenebrown.com/articles.

made it to where I am today without the benefit of a support network, which is why I remain in one to this day.

The third anchor is your food plan. The reason your food plan is particularly important in combating emotional eating is because it helps you separate your food from your feelings. Having a clear, usable food plan is *so* important during triggering and emotional situations, so that when life interrupts (and it always will), you can have confidence in knowing the food plan doesn't change. It is the single best way to maintain your sanity, because its boundaries are clear and nonnegotiable once they've been set. The food plan stays the same because life isn't going to. Think of it as putting a stake in the ground—a commitment to yourself to stay strong in your recovery when life shows up unannounced.

If you have these three anchors in place, you can stay steady when the storm comes. It takes time, and there will of course be plenty of trial and error along the way, but once these three are firmly set in place, the habit of emotional eating can be replaced with the habit of freedom. (We will dive more deeply into habits in chapter 6.)

Life is unpredictable, so it's crucial to find healthy ways to manage your feelings for all the ups and downs you will surely face. If you find yourself turning to food because of unbearable emotions, then seek help. Surround yourself with people who have been there, or with people who can help you out of there:

a therapist, a nutritionist, a trusted confidant. Find what works for you—but find it.

Similarly, once your food plan is clear as day, it no longer matters when big feelings come—and they will—because your feelings will no longer affect what you eat. An established plan takes your emotions out of the driver's seat. If the food plan is immovable, well, nothing can move it. No matter what life throws at you, you can avoid emotional eating because you'll know what to eat, as well as the best practices and strategies to implement. Food plans help create a pathway to stability and lasting, meaningful change.

SEPARATING YOUR MOOD FROM YOUR FOOD

Let me use a recent example in my own life of an extremely emotional and difficult situation that my food plan helped me get through. When my father died about three years ago, it came as a complete shock. As I prepared to go to the hospital to say goodbye, I took five minutes to throw a meal together. Some people might think that's weird. But many people had told me about the challenges of finding healthy food in a hospital setting, and it was true. I cannot stress how much having that food in my bag helped me not to worry about what I would do about food once I got there. (To be transparent, it was actually one of the few times in my life when I didn't have an appetite.)

I knew that if I *did* skip my meal because of the chaos and emotionally charged nature of the grieving process, it would make me crazy; skipping meals is a huge trigger for me, regardless of what my appetite level happens to be. As soon as I was able, I ate the lunch I had brought to the hospital, in roughly the same time window that I typically do.

After years of watching so many people navigate every variety of hardship and emotional surprise, I knew I needed to be prepared going into one of the most emotionally difficult experiences of my life. Had I gone into this situation without food, I wouldn't have been prepared and would have set myself up for a potential spiral. What's more, having this food plan in place, and therefore keeping spirals at bay, allowed me to be present to my emotional situation, painful and difficult as it was. I adored my father, and I am incredibly grateful that my food plan and preparation practices allowed me to stay present to the feelings that arose during his passing, no matter how painful.

The beauty of the food plan is that it keeps us from intertwining our life with food, and it helps us to separate our food from our mood. Even people who don't have addictive problems and tendencies use food emotionally—it's part of our culture, and the messaging for it is everywhere. But when you are committed to a routine that works for you, the possibility of abusing food emotionally is taken (wait for it . . .) off the table.

Committing to a food plan also means we *will* find ourselves being uncomfortable, and we will have to work through our feelings, big and small. All the anchors are at play in this one. With God's help and with the foundation and supports built into our food plan, we can learn to work through our feelings as they arise and ultimately learn that all feelings pass. Removing the insanity of abusing food helps us to see that we are able to face our feelings, and that doing so is better for every area of our lives. We will never grow up emotionally if we don't face our feelings—it's as simple as that.

CHAPTER 5

Spirituality

As I mentioned in the last chapter, some of these recovery concepts (including spirituality) I cover more thoroughly in my books *Satisfied* and *The Satisfied Workbook*. If you are looking for a deeper dive into this aspect of recovery, I would encourage you to look to either of these books as a companion to the spiritual journey involved in recovery that we are examining here.

I cannot emphasize enough: the battle of food addiction recovery is fought in a spiritual way. Yes, we are addressing physical experiences and habits, but at their root they are ultimately spiritual. If we don't learn to turn over our difficulties and struggles to God and let Him fight the battle, recovery will never work. We cannot fight this battle ourselves; we are already losing it. We'll never make it through without Him. Blessedly, we don't have to.

The reason I've set this concept aside as its own chapter is to drive home the importance of the need for surrender. If you are going to work the 12 Steps of Food Addiction recovery, this concept can't be reiterated enough. Your entire recovery depends on your ability to surrender control of this problem over to God. You are simply unable to do this as you are in your life right now. If your own strength were enough, you already would have been able to follow some diet or "just stop eating sugar," and you likely wouldn't be looking to this book. You've been fighting this battle for so long, and you still haven't won it. Let God take over. Only He is strong enough to bring you true freedom.

At their core, the 12 Steps are based on the understanding that we are only able to strive toward recovery because with God, all things are possible. The Bible tells us, "Abide in Me, and I in you. As the branch cannot bear fruit of itself, unless it abides in the vine, neither can you, unless you abide in Me" (John 15:4 NKJV). By abiding in God, we have access to His spirit, energy, and strength flowing through us, and therefore with Him we're able to do what we would never, ever be able to do on our own.

Think about that for a second. How encouraging to know we not only have access to the almighty God, but we also can accomplish what feels impossible through His strength and help. It can be humbling, difficult, or even painful to bring our weaknesses to God and trust Him with them, asking for His help. But doing so will lead you to abundant life and freedom.

So, what does surrendering the battle to God look like? A huge part of this process is communion with Him. An essential part of your recovery (and, frankly, your daily life) is dwelling with Him. It is absolutely necessary to spend time with Him, to sit in His presence as you learn how to allow Him to breathe through you and let His work flow through you to find the victory. Your battle is with food. Think of your time with Him (whatever form that takes) as feeding on spiritual food.

We *need* spiritual food. For many of us in our battle with food addiction, we have been feeding the wrong hunger, and with the wrong thing. Much of food addiction recovery is working toward the realization that the appetite we've been trying to feed—that hole we've been trying for so long to fill—is spiritual, which is a huge part of why we can truly "never eat enough." Physical food isn't the solution to a spiritual problem. We are looking to feed our deep-seated spiritual hunger with spiritual food.*

If you are looking for a place to start, I would encourage you to set aside some time with God (even right now) to bring your issues with food before Him in prayer. Maybe you want to

---

* Dr. Gabor Maté is an excellent resource for the spiritual and emotional components that often underlie addiction. You can find more about his incredible work at his website, www.drgabormate.com.

write down (or simply say out loud): "I'm a food addict, God, and I need Your help." You may need to bring this up to Him over and over again. I certainly do! There is so much power in surrender, in articulating our needs and struggles with God. Start here, and see what else comes up when you do. He already knows the full story but wants to hear it from you.

As with everything in your recovery journey, I encourage you not to be overwhelmed or in a hurry. These changes take time; just embracing the principle of surrender itself takes time too. No matter where you are in your relationship with God, I hope you are aware of the abundant grace you have in Him. There is no way to do this perfectly, and He has no expectation for you to do so. All He asks is that you cast your burdens on Him. He'll take care of the rest.

A steady routine of connecting with God in a dependent way—and recognizing your need for His help, love, guidance, and wisdom—is just like the food plan you are crafting for recovery. Rather than escaping life through food, you want to find engagement and true healing through communion with Him. As with all aspects of this journey, spirituality isn't one-size-fits-all. Maybe you most cherish time with God in worship. Maybe, like me, you enjoy setting aside time (perhaps in the morning before you launch into your day, or in the evening after you finish work and before you make dinner) to go on long walks and simply pray with Him, or tell Him

SPIRITUALITY

about your day and your experiences. Another great option is reading your Bible and meditating on His Word when you first wake up, to give you the proper lens and nourishment to move through the rest of your day. (My book *Satisfied* has a ninety-day plan for exactly this, if you're looking for a guidepost or plan to follow.)

This is another great opportunity to experiment with finding the routine that works best for you. There are no wrong answers here! As I've said before, the most important thing isn't finding the "right routine"—it's finding *a* routine, period. Will there be days when you don't feel like reading your Bible, or are too rushed or busy to take a prayer walk to bring your cares to Him? Of course. Life will always come bursting in. But you can learn to make time with Him a priority, regardless of life's many interruptions. Prioritize connecting with Him every day, and you'll see the results.

I'll emphasize again: So much of our recovery is about learning how to handle our feelings and not be controlled by how we feel in any given moment. A core part of healthy emotional regulation is *spiritual* regulation. If you've never embraced the type of prayer with God where you share your honest concerns and feelings, I encourage you to do so. Nothing is too big, too small, too difficult, or too pedestrian to bring to Him. He wants to hear it all. And He wants you to enjoy the peace and freedom that only He can provide.

Having the right food plan without the power to execute it isn't going to work. This process is threefold: mind, body, and spirit. We've got to address all three with equal commitment and understanding of their importance. Your recovery journey requires spiritual fitness and strength, and if you're not there currently in your spiritual life, the process of surrender will likely require time. But take heart! With God, all things are possible. Without Him, we'll only ever stay right where we started.

CHAPTER 6

Habits

Now that we've addressed the introductory steps to the mind-body-spirit triad of recovery from food addiction, it's time to look toward what all this looks like as part of your daily life. If your recovery is going to stick, you've got to think of it as cultivating a new lifestyle habit. Gone are the days of quick fixes and crash diets—we know those don't work. This food plan and recovery process is all about developing new habits that create lasting, meaningful change and result in a lifetime of freedom from food addiction.

Most people are creatures of habit. We all have our routines, our ways of doing things. Many habits we create eventually feel like second nature, as if we had no hand in forming them, even though, of course, they took conscious effort or some initial spark to put into practice. In this case, we are looking to be active participants in creating certain habits with the end goal of them feeling like second nature.

I'm sure you've heard the popular 21-Day myth at some point in your life, aka, that it takes roughly twenty-one days to build a sustainable new habit. While that may or may not be true, I want you to focus less on how quickly you can build new habits into your life and more on how to *keep them* in your life. Remember: you are building a food plan and system that works for the rest of your life, not the rest of the month.

In his best-selling book, *Atomic Habits*,[10] author James Clear offers a number of valuable insights into building good habits that are designed to create lifestyle change, not "one and done" goals (e.g., lose ten pounds on a diet). One of the basic tenets of his system is "habit stacking," which is the idea that if you build good habits into routines that are already established (aka, "stacking" them onto something that already exists), you significantly increase your chances of keeping those habits in your life. This is incredibly similar to the mindset you want to adopt: you want to build your food plan directly into your life for a lifetime of freedom from addiction. When you bear that in mind from the start, it's so much easier to keep a healthy habit.

Creating a new routine can feel challenging at first, especially when you are learning and embracing a totally new way of doing things. But once you *do* learn it, it will become the way you do it, period. A new habit, once fully adopted, becomes as automatic as any other routine in your life, like brushing your teeth or walking your dog. Your goal is to create a well-oiled machine—a habit so automatic, you can't shake it, because it's *that* integrated into your life.

HABITS AS TRANSFORMATION

Overeating recovery food plans *are* routine and structured because that helps you eliminate the "make it up as you go" approach. You want to know, every day, what your breakfast, lunch, and dinner are going to be (and what each meal is made up of) so you don't have to think about food throughout your day. Keeping your plan simple and clear is hugely important in limiting triggers and one of the best ways to enhance success in your recovery. It's much easier to follow a plan that you know works for you when you don't have a lot to trip you up. As food addicts, most of us are all too familiar with playing with our food: "I'll just have one cookie," "I can always eat more vegetables at dinner to make up for this whole bag of chips," and so on. When you have a food plan that you know works, you stand a better chance of stopping these thought spirals in their tracks and sticking to a freedom-focused path. You throw out an old habit that created confusion and replace it with a new habit that keeps you focused on your recovery.

On the other end of the spectrum, a food plan also helps eliminate the damaging "counting" or "points" aspects that so many diets tout. When we are constantly doing the math of each new diet we try, it's easy to get discouraged, become obsessed with hitting "the right mark," or simply become overwhelmed (which itself is a huge trigger for many). We want to replace that thinking with a focus on the appropriate ratios of proteins, vegetables, starches, and fats that you can craft on your plate at any given meal, for delight and satisfaction and freedom from confusion. The plug-and-play formula of the Satisfied Food Plan functions so that it's easy to remember and use in any given context (which we'll get into more in later chapters). Once you've got it down, you can incorporate it into all your meals without much work or thought. It'll be as routine as flossing.

Let's look at an example to put all this into context. Let's say you're a woman, and you've done your trial and error to figure out your food plan. You've found that, at each meal, the best food balance involves three ounces of protein, a tablespoon of fat, a serving of vegetables, and a grain of some kind. Having discovered this, you can plug in the foods that work best for you based on this simple formula, and switch things up whenever you like, based on taste and preference. One day at lunch, you have salad as your vegetable; the next day you enjoy broccoli. The food itself matters less than knowing you're getting your vegetable. Or, if having the same food is a way to maintain sanity for you, you can simply eat the same meals on varying rotations that fit the plan criteria.

The most important thing is that you keep the routine—the habit—that you've found works for you. The goal behind the effort and experimenting is to eventually arrive at a personalized plan that you are so good at, you no longer have to think about it. We are after *automatic*. Again, I know a lot of this seems overwhelming at first, but you'll be surprised at how instinctive it can become when you embrace the recovery journey with all of your mind, body, and spirit.

We are not looking to reinvent the wheel. We already know that doesn't work for us. So many of us have looked to fad diets or hot new regimens peddled by diet culture promising that if we "just eat this" or "just cut out that" we will finally look the way we want and stop craving *x*, *y*, or *z*. We all know how that turns out.

With your food plan, you are after *simplicity*. The goal is to have a straightforward plan and then stick to it, so much so that it becomes second nature. Variety can certainly come into play inside the parameters of your plan, but the system itself doesn't change. You're done with that. Instead of the confusion and desperation that often come from not having a plan in place, you'll have habits that allow you to make sensible decisions for yourself.

HABITS AS PATHWAYS

As we discussed in chapter 2, our brains have been hijacked in the past by all the junk food we have consumed. Our pathways have told us that the dopamine we have historically gotten from binge eating means we need to constantly be eating more and more junk food to stay "happy."* That has been our habit. The food plan is part of retraining your brain. You want your pathways to take you to places of satiety and nourishment so that your body is back to a regulated place where sustainable health is possible. It takes some time, but once you've retrained your brain, it all gets easier. It's just like driving—you don't have to look up the directions to places you regularly go to, because you already know how to get there. That's how second nature this will become, if you commit to this lifestyle change.

Outside of learning the proper ratios and portions for our respective food plans (the nuts and bolts of which we'll get into later), we've got to build proper lifestyle and spiritual habits

---

* It's easy to conflate dopamine and serotonin. They are very similar. Both are considered "happy" chemicals; both are neurotransmitters in the brain. According to the Cleveland Clinic, dopamine is the chemical associated with rewards and motivation—for our purposes, the "reward" that has gotten further out of reach with each binge; serotonin is more generally associated with "happy feelings." (See "What's the Difference between Dopamine and Serotonin?" Cleveland Clinic, March 18, 2022, https://my.clevelandclinic.org/health/articles/22572-serotonin.)

into our lives as well. We need to make sure our mental health is in order, just like our physical health. We got into this a bit in the last chapter, but it bears repeating. Every day, we need to have healthy habits in place for our spirituality and our mental health. Whether that's daily quiet time, scheduled connection to a recovery group, podcasts that inspire, or some combination of these things—each of us must build habits into our life that keep us healthy in every aspect. We need encouragement and accountability every step of the way.

One facet of maintaining overall wellness is addressing emotional strife as it comes up.* As we've already talked about, most of us have turned to food to stuff whatever emotions we are experiencing. This is another habit we want to replace with something that can become second nature and, even more important, help us deal with our emotions responsibly and healthily. For instance, a habit you could build into your life would be journaling whenever you experience painful feelings, or making a quick phone call to a friend, or finding a therapist to help you parse through those feelings. Some of this will certainly feel uncomfortable after so many years of stuffing things down with food. Repetition is key; you must commit to

---

* Again, I encourage you to check out Dr. Gabor Maté; he is a proponent of "compassionate inquiry" into the underlying issues of addiction. His work is an invaluable, life-changing resource.

the practices you want to build into your life in order to keep them there.

Overall, we have a lifetime of bad habits surrounding both food and lifestyle that we are looking to root out and replace with sustainable, healthy habits that keep us on the path toward freedom and recovery. Again, these are long-term strategies for long-term success, not another empty promise of "thirty days to a new you." Dealing with your emotions is difficult! Committing to a new way of doing things is difficult. Creating new habits is difficult. These things take time, energy, patience, and trust in something you can't quite see yet. It's a tall order, and it's no joke! But habits are the key. Habits are the mainstays, the things we lean on when we are tossed by the storms of life. Once we plug space into our days to accomplish the habits we need to establish food freedom, we *will* see results.

Over the years, food has taken up so much of our lives and time—much more time and energy than it will take to build these new healthy practices to make our lives manageable and livable. This may sound cliché, but it's so true: it's the journey, not the destination. Once these habits become as easy to us as driving to work or taking our vitamins, we will be so much safer around food and back to living our lives again. The time that we lost will be redeemed, and so much of what we thought we had lost forever to addiction will be restored to abundance. If that's not worth the effort, I don't know what is.

CHAPTER 7

Planning and Preparing— Give Up Excuses and Make Up Your Mind

As I'm sure you are starting to understand this far into the book, recovery is multifaceted and affects every area of your life. Yes, it's a lifestyle change, but it's also a straight-up *life* change to embrace and commit to food recovery. All of what we've talked about falls under one big umbrella necessary for everything to shift: your mindset. Without a mindset shift, nothing can really change or fall into place. It's time to get serious about your commitment to recovery and finally eating well.

While this is obviously part of my story, it needs to become part of yours too: planning meals and prepping food is essential to successfully changing a lifestyle. Yes, your process will by no means be perfect or picturesque, but the commitment must be constant. Think about it this way: If you had cancer, you wouldn't forget to go to your cancer treatment. If you were a diabetic, you would take your insulin. Food addiction is equally detrimental, so you must take the consequences and fallout seriously.

Continuing to mess around with food means continuing to mess around with your life, based on the damage caused by an eating disorder (or food addiction). Following a pattern of chaos and confusion keeps you focused on food and weight instead of your peace. It keeps you in the battle. Our whole lives are stunted when we don't take our recovery seriously. And *that's* why it's so critical to commit to crafting a food plan, and to a mind, body, and spirit change. It's imperative to do so to bring your life back into balance, and to finally find peace. It's the only way out of the hole that our lives have fallen into.

For some of us, it's easy to not care about ourselves. Many habits (like those we're trying to eradicate and replace, as we talked about in the previous chapter) are ones of self-neglect, laziness, even despondency. Our addiction has taken over our whole lives, and our habits and patterns are in accordance with that. We've checked out completely; we feel like giving up. Some of us may even be at the point where we no longer want to live. I know I certainly felt that way at my lowest point, because I just couldn't see a way out of the cyclone of chaos.

PLANNING AND PREPARING—GIVE UP EXCUSES AND MAKE UP YOUR MIND

Others of us have doctors telling us that if we don't modify our eating and our health habits, things will only get worse: heart attack and disease, diabetes, and so on.* Some of us may already be in incredibly poor health and suffering from these very conditions. When looked at through this sobering lens, your recovery really is a matter of life and death. Shouldn't you treat it that way?

The end goal of keeping you alive and well is a lot different from losing ten pounds or "looking thin." What's more, from a spiritual perspective, it's learning to take care of your body as a temple unto God, and rejecting the old ways of abusing and neglecting it. We need a whole new way of looking at things.

PREPARATION IS KEY

A huge part of your overall treatment is your eating plan and the necessary preparation that comes once you commit to following it. I'll keep saying it until it's tattooed on your brain: your food plan is essential to shutting down the insanity. You've got to update your mindset from food being a source of emotional comfort, or fear, or confusion—whatever it has represented in your life up to this point—and start viewing

---

* You've already heard me say this, but Dr. Mark Hyman has a true gift for breaking down the physical (and mental) side effects of not eating correctly. I encourage you to check out his work at www.drhyman.com.

food as a source of nourishment, as a crucial way of taking care of your body and yourself as an anchor in the recovery process. Food is not the enemy—*abusing* food is. This will be a huge mindset shift for many of us.

As we touched on in the last chapter, a major mindset change brings many new habits that may feel unfamiliar as we begin embracing them. With a new manual for life comes all kinds of new rules; we can't look to old habits or patterns if we want new, lasting results and change. You might feel overwhelmed at the prospect, but take heart: change is built one day at a time, and you don't have to tackle everything all at once. You've just got to be willing to start.

For instance, as you commit to your food plan, you'll put a major habit into place: going to the grocery store every week and filling your cupboards and fridge with only what's nourishing and already on your plan. If you want to be successful, set yourself up for success. That means not having anything in the house that can trip you up or throw you right back to where you started. Which, in turn, means making a grocery list before you go to the store that you commit to sticking to, no matter what starts calling your name in aisle seven.

For many of us, this isn't just a mindset change—it's a whole *schedule* change. Cooking your food at home (therefore taking the time to plan your meals, shop for them, and then

PLANNING AND PREPARING—GIVE UP EXCUSES AND MAKE UP YOUR MIND

actually prep and make them) is a significant time commitment for many people, especially if your food addiction has involved a lot of takeout and processed, grab-and-go food. At the beginning, it may also feel like a whole new financial landscape: paying more for healthier food rather than cheaper, faster options. That said, grocery shopping and cooking for yourself consistently is actually much more cost effective than regularly eating out; the bill is simply larger at one time instead of being split into smaller amounts of money at every meal. Again, it's a *lifestyle* change—committing to doing this for real is going to affect all areas of your life.

Maybe thinking about lifestyle changes is stirring some feelings and reactions in you: "I don't want to spend the money. I can't take all that time to plan and shop ahead of time. This sounds like too much work."

Please hear me when I say: These are just feelings. And many of these feelings have kept you in addiction, simply eating based on emotions and avoiding the hard work of recovery by taking the easy way out. You are setting yourself up for failure if you don't develop a consistent practice that keeps you eating well and healthy as opposed to eating what you feel like, when you feel like it. With that mindset, you simply end up at the drive-thru eating fast food, falling back into old toxic habits, because you don't have what you already need in your house, waiting to be made.

NO MORE EXCUSES

It's time to learn to stop making excuses. To do so, we've got to get back to basics; we are doing a full rewiring of the system. If you have always believed that healthy food is gross or that it takes too much work to prepare or that you're not good at cooking, I would encourage you to be open to a new way of doing things. Because the bottom line is this: it's just as easy to eat healthy food as it is to eat unhealthy food. It's simply a matter of learning how to do it well and in a way that works for your life.

For instance, your meal prep can be as easy as ordering a healthy delivery service. What's more, the internet is an invaluable resource for thousands of easy, fast recipes right at your fingertips that won't send you spiraling. If work or home life takes up the bulk of your day and you find yourself short on time, seek out an option that doesn't take as long. If you *have* time to cook but are averse to it, find recipes that are easy and short to start with and see how they might change your attitude. Just take it one step at a time. Commit to trying a new aspect of what is required, and build on more each week.

Our excuses are just that—excuses. Are some of these feelings valid? Absolutely. Will it take significant effort and time to change? You bet. But again, I want you to think about these things as changing your entire mindset around food and

PLANNING AND PREPARING—GIVE UP EXCUSES AND MAKE UP YOUR MIND

your problems with it. I want to encourage you to set aside whatever excuses are plaguing you and to think of yourself as a person in treatment for a serious problem. Taking care of and treating yourself is like any other condition that needs care: If you're sick, you take medicine. If your grass is too long, you mow it.

Maybe you're in an emotional place right now where you don't feel worthy of good treatment or respect, and you can't fathom the thought of taking care of yourself. First, let me just say: You are worthy of care. You are worthy of freedom. The God of the universe thought you were worth dying for, and He loves and cares for you more than you could ever imagine. If you don't see yourself this way—if this is a familiar excuse or outdated mindset that's keeping you stuck in old patterns of addiction—then imagine all this as treatment for someone you care about deeply, like a family member or friend. If they were truly, life-threateningly sick, wouldn't you encourage them to do everything in their power and resources to get well?

As intense as this sounds, it's also important to remember that not everything about this lifestyle change has to feel sobering and serious. You have so much room to have fun with these new habits and patterns. Maybe that can include a habit you're trying to "stack" into all this: gratitude and joy. Maybe it means turning on some of your favorite music while you cook, and treating however long it takes to prepare your meal like your personal dance party. Maybe your weekly grocery shopping is the time you carve out to call a friend you love and trust. If you can find a way to plan and prepare food that you like, you just might find that it's not a burden after all. It's all about how you frame it.

MAKE UP YOUR MIND

As we know by now, it takes some dedicated time and effort to readjust your perspective and, ultimately, change your life—but the bottom line is it's what's required. To break the cycle of addiction that you are stuck in, you need a full perspective shift. It takes as long as it takes, and it requires a willingness to keep at it even when it's hard and you can't quite understand what's happening (or if it's helping). You've got to trust God and the recovery process, and lean into Him when despair or discouragement threaten to throw you off course. With God's help, you are committing to crafting and sticking to a healthy, sustainable plan and to stocking your home with only the foods that fall under its guidelines so that they are ready to eat when you need them.

So how do you put the mindset change into practice? First, I encourage you to take stock of your life to see what habits and patterns can be most successfully built in as you learn how to change. For instance, if you have to leave early in the morning

PLANNING AND PREPARING—GIVE UP EXCUSES AND MAKE UP YOUR MIND

for work, I highly recommend doing advance food preparation for the week. Think of it as self-care, an "appointment" in your wellness regimen, a gift to future you from present you. One option is doing batch cooking over the weekend, at a time that works best for you, and prepping all of your food for the week so you'll have fast, easy meals ready when you need to run out the door. Again, think of this time and effort as removing the possibility of lapsing—that's the goal. Not weight loss, not emotional avoidance—freedom from addiction and removal of temptation. You're not going to get it perfect right away. But you *will* gradually build new habits into your life, so you don't end up with the same results you've had up to this point.

Second, make up your mind and then state your intention clearly. It might help to tell yourself, *I am going to have what I need in my pantry on hand, and I will follow a food plan that supports and keeps me in my recovery. I won't leave my house without the food I need, or without a plan for how I'm going to eat for the day.* Be honest with yourself, find what works for you, and then stick to it. You can break it down into manageable chunks along the way; the process won't fall magically together overnight.

Third, it's equally important to make sure the food you incorporate into your food plan tastes good! So many of us have believed our whole lives that healthy food can't taste good. I know I felt that way; the only vegetables I ate growing up came out of a can, and I dreaded when they were on the menu at dinnertime. But that was just another excuse I had to let go of as I embraced the new mindset, and the same is true for you. Healthy food *can* and *does* taste good! You've just got to take some time to find out what you like after so many years of eating highly processed foods like french fries and pizza because that's what was convenient. Or maybe you never learned how to properly prepare healthy food. As you reset and begin exploring the nuts and bolts of the foods you'll incorporate into your plan, be willing to experiment and try new things. Maybe embrace a type of cooking you've never tried before, or prepare a dish using a seasoning you normally wouldn't use.

If the thought of that totally turns you off, don't be afraid to seek help. Maybe consider hiring a nutritionist, or ask an employee at the grocery store what prepackaged veggie or other healthy meal options they have. You could also ask a recovery buddy to come with you to provide insight and support—someone who gets the recovery process and the level of care you need to take when food shopping. There are so many resources you can look to and so many opportunities to turn this lifestyle change into something you enjoy and look forward to. Asking for help might look like inviting a friend who's a good cook over for dinner and making something together.

Many of us have spent too much time in the isolation that food addiction breeds. But I'll say it again: you are *not* alone in your recovery. So many people have walked this path before you, and all kinds of support awaits you if you just take that first step toward changing your mindset. It's work, but that doesn't mean you can't have fun along the way!

Through all this, I encourage you to be daring and to explore outside your comfort zone. There's that word again: *comfort*.* For so long, many of us have looked to food for comfort when things got hard or didn't immediately feel easy. That's an old, meager habit; we want to instead bring in the abundant and new. You don't have to keep doing what you've always done once you make up your mind that it isn't working for you. There's a whole new world of freedom and deliciousness to explore. Doesn't that sound so much better than the craziness and confusion of food addiction?

---

* Once again, Brené Brown is an excellent resource in the emotional landscape of getting outside your comfort zone—and the rewards that await on the other side. Her book *Daring Greatly* is a great place to start if you are not already familiar with her work.

Quick Tips from Dr. Rhona: Ideas for Easy Bites

Do you sometimes need a quick meal or snack that's ready on the go? Part 3 will include some recipes to try, but in the meantime, here are some easy, healthy alternatives to fast food. Just start by including the necessities in your weekly grocery run so that they're ready to go.

- Veggie burger with a prewashed salad mix and fruit
- Precooked salmon or rotisserie chicken with a side of your favorite veggies (check local grocery store for precooked options)
- Ezekiel English muffin with almond butter and (unsweetened) fruit spread, with fruit
- Organic chicken hot dog in a brown-rice wrap with a prewashed salad mix
- Ground chicken (browned) with spinach and brown rice, or chickpea pasta with seasonings and (sugar-free) tomato or pesto sauce
- Bagged salad mix with precooked chicken added
- Pre-made brown rice bowl with veggies and protein
- Healthy frozen-meal delivery services

CHAPTER 8

Backup Plans — Restaurants and Vacations

I hope you're beginning to feel motivated and hopeful about the freedom that's in store once you embrace the many aspects of recovery we've talked about so far. Maybe you're even starting to see that it *is* possible to find freedom from the craziness of food addiction, and that sanity is within reach once you begin addressing the root problems.

A lot of what we've discussed has had to do with changing your routines and habits, as well as learning how to craft a food plan that works for your lifestyle based on your needs and preferences. In this chapter, we're going to look at how to approach situations that fall outside the norm, like vacations and parties, and discuss strategies for the times you're not at home in your own kitchen.

First of all, it's important to remember that your concern in any given scenario isn't "breaking a diet"—it's breaking your recovery. You want the idea of *mindset*—which we looked at in chapter 7—to permeate every area of your life. As I go through some examples of "life interruptions" where you'll need to have a plan, remember that one lapse for a food addict can set us back much more than a day—it can lead to a total backslide from any progress up to that point. It's just not the same as a "cheat day" or "falling off the wagon." You want ways to move through life that keep you on the path to freedom, and joyfully so. You'll have to find new ways to navigate various situations, but when you approach them with the new mindset of embracing recovery, doing so becomes much more straightforward and sustainable.

As with everything in the recovery process, the beginning is the hardest, when temptation is at an all-time high. Family gatherings, restaurants, or weekly coffee shop meetups with a friend—you've got to reassess what going to these places looks like now that you are in recovery and have a different mindset.

If it's possible, I would encourage you to give yourself time away from old places while you're establishing your food plan at home. Take some time to get your spiritual and emotional health in check, so you can approach going to restaurants and gatherings with a stronger resolve. If one of your goals is to deal healthily with your emotions,* it's a good idea to allow time to develop those skills before putting yourself in a situation where you might be tempted to go off the deep end. If you have the option to take this retreat at the outset of your recovery process, communicate these boundaries to your family and friends.† Let them know you need some time, and maybe ask if they're open, for a while, to other ways of meeting and connecting that don't involve food. Ask members of your support group how they have navigated these situations. Help yourself be prepared so that when these situations arise (and they will), you'll have all kinds of strategies at your disposal.

EMBRACING DISCOMFORT

Whether you can take some time to reset or not, you will, like all of us, face some uncomfortable situations where you're no longer able to eat what you used to eat with other people. For example, maybe you're part of a family that regularly eats fast food. Let's say you're on a road trip, and you know everyone

---

* Reminder: Dr. Gabor Maté's "compassionate inquiry" approach is an excellent place to start if you are looking to begin developing healthy "emotional muscles."
† In her book *Good Boundaries and Goodbyes,* Lysa TerKeurst provides practical, real-life strategies and examples for implementing boundaries in your relationships—even the ones that feel impossible.

will want to grab fast food for dinner. You've got a couple of options here. One, since you know this is your family's way of doing things, pack yourself a dinner before you head out so you have something in the car and won't have to worry about it. Will this feel inconvenient at first? Possibly. It might mean an independent trip to the grocery store during (if not before) your trip, and setting aside extra time to do so. But a little inconvenience is a lot better than ending up not having what you need, and being in a position where the only food available is highly processed and full of addictive ingredients. Remember: the motivating force behind these new habits is that you are building a life that strengthens your recovery.

Another option is to ask your family if they're willing to stop somewhere that has options for everyone. This doesn't mean forcing your new lifestyle on the people in your life. It just means you're asking for what you need. Think back on times when a friend or loved one asked for something they needed; how did you and others respond? You might be surprised at how willingly the people who love you will help you on your journey.

Maybe you're shaking your head right now because those options don't seem possible. Don't be discouraged; asking for what you need and asserting yourself can certainly be difficult, and a lot of us aren't in a place where we can do that quite yet. It's a skill we are likely learning in tandem with all the other

BACKUP PLANS—RESTAURANTS AND VACATIONS

aspects of our recovery, after so many years of quieting our needs by stuffing them down with food, often in total isolation and out of sight from the people we love. Many of us have been accustomed to people-pleasing to get through our lives. But people-pleasing can sabotage us. And remember, we are looking at food addiction through the mindset of any other life-threatening illness. If you were an alcoholic, and everyone else around you were drinking, you wouldn't drink. Similarly, if everyone in your family is eating highly processed fast food, and you're addicted to that, you're not going to eat it. And it will be a whole lot easier to stick to that if you use one of the strategies I mentioned. It is now your responsibility to prepare ahead of time. No one else will do it for you!

Relationships are complex, and difficult family dynamics are often why some of us turned to food addiction in the first place. Everyone's journey and experience is different. I encourage you to get comfortable knowing that others might not understand the reality of food addiction. It can be a particularly touchy subject in many relationships, because regardless of how you present it, when you share that you need an alternative option to eat, it's easy for others to think you are telling *them* that how *they're* eating is "wrong." (Of course, it's important that we express our needs in a personal way with no hint of questioning anyone else's choices.) You are the best judge of how to bring this up with the people in your life. As long as you respect your addiction and take the reality of it seriously, nobody else needs to—though, of course, it certainly is a huge help when we receive support from others.

ALWAYS HAVE A PLAN

Either way, no matter your circumstances—and no matter where you find yourself—like everything else we've been learning up to this point, you always, always, *always* have to have a plan. For instance, if a friend asks you to meet for dinner at a local restaurant, look up the menu ahead of time and figure out what will work for you and what won't. When doing this, focus on what you *can* eat, not what you *can't*. In this day and age, most places have healthy options that are yummy and that we can enjoy with our loved ones. Take the time to make sure you aren't going to a place where you can't eat anything. If there aren't any options, again, I would encourage you to ask if you could meet somewhere else, and suggest a place you know works for you (and your friend). If you don't have that type of relationship (or if it's for a special occasion like a birthday party, where it's not appropriate for you to pick the place), it might mean saying no and sitting that particular social gathering out, or eating ahead of time and committing to just enjoying company at the restaurant.

On that note, you should start getting comfortable saying no to certain gatherings until you confidently know that being there won't throw off your recovery. Again, this will likely be more difficult at the outset; but the stronger you become emotionally and spiritually, and the more you surround yourself with support and encouragement, the easier it will get. It won't always feel like a "thing" every time you go out.

Another muscle we're learning to exercise and strengthen in our recovery is how to do our own thing in any given situation. If you're comfortable being in a restaurant environment again, and everyone you're with is sharing plates, you will likely have to order your own separate dish. Sure, this might feel awkward the first few times, but try to bear in mind the reality of your recovery. Think about your decisions in these circumstances in terms of how you will feel about them after you leave and go home. It's not worth conforming to social pressure for an evening if it sends you home to a binge spiral that nobody sees.

WHAT ABOUT VACATION?

One of the biggest questions I get from my clients in food recovery is, "What do I do when I'm on vacation?" For many people, vacation is a time to forgo normal routines and let loose. One of the biggest areas where most people apply this is, unsurprisingly, food. It's easy to equate vacation as a time of indulgence, when "calories don't count"; when what happens on vacation—and what is eaten on vacation—stays on vacation. But addiction doesn't take a vacation, ever.

And so I'm going to tell you what I've told my clients throughout the years: no matter your destination, no matter who you're with, no matter how you feel—staying on plan is more important. You want to be able to return from vacation with your sanity intact. Do whatever you must to have your food figured out ahead of time. Sometimes that means packing nonperishables to enjoy while there. It might look like making the grocery store your first stop on vacation, and doing a bit of research ahead of time to find one that suits your needs near. When I travel, I almost always order delivery from a local grocery store to coincide with my arrival, so my food is waiting at my destination. There are myriad ways to follow your plan wherever you are. Once you get the hang of it, even though you're on vacation, it'll have that same "second nature" quality of any other routine. You'll be able to enjoy your vacation and relax in knowing that you're not going to be at the mercy of temptations and potential slip-ups.

ASK FOR WHAT YOU NEED

While you're figuring out all these situations and scenarios, it's important to develop your new habits with support. Don't try to do this in isolation! Take advantage of the resources at

BACKUP PLANS—RESTAURANTS AND VACATIONS

your disposal. Set up a meeting with your sponsor before you agree to meet a friend out or prior to a vacation. Ask people in your recovery group what they suggest doing, and be honest about your need for encouragement. Food addiction is about isolation and feeling like nobody else could possibly understand your situation. Recovery is about embracing community and finding healing in knowing you're not alone and that other people have been exactly where you are.

Also, let's be clear: it can be really hard to be around people who are indulging in food! I had to say no to many social gatherings while I was establishing my recovery, because it was just plain *too hard* for me to be around the foods that made me crazy at the start. I knew it was too much of a temptation, so I had to take my time to sort out my heart and spirit so I could be with the people I loved without my food fixations taking over. I have put a lot of work into shifting my mindset to the things that I can indulge in that are good for me: indulging in connecting with the people that I'm with at a restaurant; indulging in some extra time with God to help get my mind right before a stressful situation where a trigger may be present; indulging in a walk in nature when I start to feel discouraged.

It might sound improbable to you now, but it is amazing how your life starts to change when you lean more deeply into all the areas food was holding you hostage. Once you've put food in its proper place and know that you have a good plan for any situation, you can really *be* with the people you're with, wherever you are.

    There are so many more wonderful things to indulge in other than junk food, and none of them will leave you feeling hopeless and trapped. So often when we abused food, we were looking for something food could never provide: love, safety, connection, joy. All these things are available in good fellowship and relationship with God and the people we love. What's more, they're available to us the more we connect with our recovery groups or our therapists, or just talk on the phone with a friend who *gets* it. It's a different mindset, and that takes time to develop. Nobody gets this stuff right the first time, and every new day brings a new situation that we have to learn how to navigate. You are exercising new muscles in your heart and your head. And every time you do, you guarantee a better chance at long-term success in your recovery journey.

BACKUP PLANS—RESTAURANTS AND VACATIONS

Quick Tips from Dietitian Jackie: 10 Ideas for Enjoying Restaurants with Friends and Family

1. When looking at the menu, focus on the heart-healthy or health-conscious options. These foods are typically grilled or steamed, making them a safe and healthy option.
2. Eating at a restaurant often involves sharing appetizers or entrees. If the selections don't work with your plan, explain that you're on a special plan and it's best that you order your own separate option.
3. When placing an order, immediately request a take-home box, so you are able to pack up the excess portion of your dish for another meal and prevent overeating.
4. Always ask for dressings, condiments, or sauces on the side to control the amount you use.

5. When selecting a side dish, pick a healthy selection such as fruit or vegetables, or decline altogether.
6. Avoiding buffets and complimentary food items like bread or chips is difficult. In order to avoid them, let your server know you'd like to pass on any complimentary items.
7. Just because the menu says it's a "healthy choice" doesn't necessarily mean it's the right choice for your plan.
8. Avoid foods that say *fried*, *crunchy*, or *crispy*; these items are typically breaded and fried, which can be triggering.
9. Ordering two appetizers rather than an entree is a good way to control your portion size while giving yourself some variety.
10. When it comes to dessert, order a hot beverage like coffee or tea. This way you can partake in ordering something while avoiding those trigger foods.

CHAPTER 9

Parties, Holidays, and Catered Affairs

This chapter is similar to the previous one in that it deals with situations that fall outside the norm of your routine. I've chosen to separate the two because this one deals with more specialized circumstances over which, compared to vacations, you may have less control—such as parties and catered affairs in personal and professional situations. No matter what circumstance you find yourself in, I want to help you have a plan for it to keep your recovery strong.

As I've worked with people over the years in my counseling practice, I've learned that the situations we'll be looking at in this chapter can push people's buttons when they're in recovery for a variety of reasons. I have helped them find ways to navigate all kinds of events, and I'm confident that this chapter will help you do the same. You've got to take things one day at a time, but I promise: these scenarios will get easier the longer you are in recovery. It's all part of using that new mindset we're learning to cultivate and exercising the developing muscles that our addiction has weakened.

PARTIES

To state the obvious: no one wants to feel like the odd one out or the downer at a party! We want to participate in what everyone else is doing, not feel like we're being needy or a bother to our friends or the host. Food addicts tend to be people pleasers, or we simply don't want to draw additional attention to ourselves. We've got to recognize that from the start so we don't stuff down that feeling while we're looking for ways to keep our recovery going.

What's more, in a party setting, most of us don't want people to know we have a problem, so we don't want to say anything about it. We'd rather fly under the radar and go with the flow. It certainly feels much easier to go along with whatever food is there and to do whatever everyone else is doing. But remember: things are different now. We are in recovery, and so we've got to learn appropriate ways to address situations where we *do* need an alternate way of doing things, without disrupting experiences for others.

PARTIES, HOLIDAYS, AND CATERED AFFAIRS

Let's take a look at catered affairs, such as a business meeting or wedding. Obviously, the relationships involved in these examples differ (professional versus personal), but many of the underlying principles and strategies translate well to either. For both events, a caterer is typically involved, meaning your point of contact for any questions about what food will be prepared is somewhat removed from the situation. The food is often neither in your control nor the host's, meaning you're going to have to do a bit more detective work than when you're just meeting a friend out for dinner, like we discussed in the previous chapter.

When possible, I recommend finding out in advance what the food at an event like this is going to be. That might mean shooting the host a text to find out who's catering, or looking at the event invitation to see what information is available about the food. It's typically easier to track down the caterer than you might think. Once you have that info, simply contact the caterer and ask about the menu and what possibilities are available for someone with different food needs. In most cases, you can ask for what you need; caterers are accustomed to those kinds of requests. Stuff like this is no different than calling ahead about a food allergy, especially when you ask in advance. When you ask ahead, it means the host or caterer *can* prepare you something in advance. When you don't, you have to figure it out on the fly, and we know by now that's something we're looking to avoid.

Does that mean that when you plan ahead you're always going to have your first choice available? Of course not. You've got to get flexible, and sometimes you'll have to roll with the punches and take what's available. That might mean just oil and vinegar for your salad if the only other option is a sweet creamy dressing. Remember: our goal is no longer keeping a diet or counting calories against cheat days. The question we are always asking is: "What do I have to do in order to sustain my recovery?"

Whatever questions you need to ask at events like these, there's typically a way to do so discreetly so as not to draw attention to yourself or take away from the event itself. If it's an event with staff, like a wedding, let the server (or a member of the catering team) know you're the one who called ahead about a special meal. They'll know what to do—another great bonus of making sure everything is taken care of ahead of time.

If the staff presses you and asks what your food allergies are, tell them exactly what you need: "Can you provide me with a meal that's just plain chicken and vegetables without all the sauces and breading?" You don't need to explain *why* you need a special meal. You don't owe anyone a reason for your needs, and you don't have to share the specifics. You can advocate for yourself. I know you may feel awkward trying this the first few times, but in my experience, both for myself and

PARTIES, HOLIDAYS, AND CATERED AFFAIRS

the people I've treated, it's the best way to get what you need: simply asking for it.

Conversely, if you're going to a more casual event, like a party at a friend's house, don't be afraid to text ahead and ask what's being served. Be clear: you're not asking them to *prepare* something for you! You're just trying to get all the information to make the best plan for yourself, so you'd like to know what'll be there for your specific dietary restrictions. You can even offer to bring something for yourself. It doesn't have to be a whole ordeal, and you'll get better at it as you go.

Once you get the hang of it, it's much easier to ask for what you need, and you'll feel like a pro navigating these circumstances. You'll also learn that, more often than not, people want to help you when they can. Especially people who love you. But you have to be the most willing to help yourself, because it's your responsibility to make sure your food needs are taken care of. No one else is going to manage your recovery but you. No matter the event, you have to go home with *you* when it's over. So you want to be happy with yourself, and you don't want to be set up for a spiral of anxiety or confusion because you didn't ask for what you needed ahead of time.

Ultimately, people-pleasing just isn't worth it when you look at what's at stake. As we've discussed, there's a way to do these things politely and discreetly. You're not being a bother when you ask for what you need. You are taking care of yourself and maintaining your recovery.

To help you work through the uncomfortable feelings that may arise when you're trying these things out, focus on the purpose of the event: the fun itself and the people you're celebrating with. See if there are ways to be helpful to your host or fellow guests. Once you've got your needs taken care of, you can shift your focus from the food that could be tempting or troubling to the many other things you can celebrate and enjoy. When you look for ways to be a blessing, you'll find how much better every experience is. I'm certain it'll leave you feeling much more satisfied and grateful.

HOLIDAYS

Finally, let's take a look at holidays. I know we touched on this in the last chapter, but now it's time to go a bit deeper into the many little minefields you may find yourself encountering at holiday gatherings. This is a big one for most of my clients, because holidays can bring up a range of emotions for a variety of reasons, so they are often more complicated to deal with and require more specificity. This is a huge area where many of us can get trapped, and I want to help you as much as I can to not feel that way.

It bears repeating: our addiction doesn't take a break just because it's Christmas (or Thanksgiving). It's so tempting to

PARTIES, HOLIDAYS, AND CATERED AFFAIRS

slip into that "vacation mindset" we talked about in the last chapter. It's also easy, especially during the holidays, to get nostalgic for all kinds of food traditions we've indulged in over the years. For many of us, it feels impossible to even imagine the holidays without certain foods, like pumpkin pie at Thanksgiving or our grandmother's Yule log cake at the family Christmas gathering. We all have foods we feel attached to during the holiday seasons, foods that we associate or even equate with the holiday itself.

I know so many people who have lost their recovery at a holiday gathering—sometimes more than once. As noted previously, for us there is no "I'll just have a piece of pie." That simply isn't how it works for food addicts. This isn't a cheat meal or a "deserved treat." We've got to rewire all that messaging we've taken in from diet culture over the years. We know what will happen if we just have "one piece." We've already walked that road. If you find yourself feeling nostalgic about food-based traditions, I'd gently remind you about all that came with indulging them: chaos, bingeing, woe. We are walking a new road now, one we know won't leave us raiding our fridge in the middle of the night or going off the deep end.

You won't be surprised to hear me say that the biggest thing you can do for yourself is to plan ahead. If that means eating your whole meal at home before going to your family's Thanksgiving, do what you have to do. Or you can certainly bring your own healthy dish for everyone to enjoy, and for most holiday meals you have a good understanding of what foods will be available that won't break your recovery. It's easy to feel triggered or emotional based on our family's reactions to any requests we might make or have, but that's part of the emotional terrain we're learning to navigate. It takes time, but you are learning. I believe in you!

A big part of our recovery, specifically around holidays and family gatherings, is shifting the focus away from the food to everything else that the holidays are about: relationships, gratitude, time set aside to connect and celebrate with people we love. When this concept shifts from being abstract to concrete, you'll be surprised at how quiet those crazy-making voices in your head can become. It takes practice and work, but as your mindset changes, so will your patience and ability.

There are all kinds of ways to still participate in family holiday gatherings in your recovery, even if they take some getting used to. A lot of this can sound like depriving yourself, but it's just a different, healthier way of enjoying yourself with people you love. While everyone else is having dessert, maybe you can make yourself a yummy cup of tea or pack some fruit to enjoy on your own. Maybe you can use this time where others are indulging in food to go for a walk and take some time with God, or offer to help someone else clean up, or start a meaningful conversation with a relative you haven't seen in a

PARTIES, HOLIDAYS, AND CATERED AFFAIRS

long time. Look for opportunities to fill up on the things your soul is actually hungry for: connection, love, gratitude.

As you develop these new habits, you'll learn to love the holidays for what they're ultimately about, not the food that traditionally comes with them. You've got to stick with your food plan year-round, because you are a food addict year-round. Other people who don't deal with this addiction can gain a few extra pounds over the holidays, but they can also stop after a bit of indulgence. It's just not the case with food addicts.

Sure, there might be some room to relax a bit in your food plan during the holidays, but that is something to think through in advance. You've got to take your time through the process, and make room for things being more difficult at the beginning. Once your food plan and boundaries are clearly established and you've had some good practice, maybe you have a heartier meal than usual during your Thanksgiving dinner, or enjoy some fruit you don't normally have. The food plan is designed with flexibility in mind, but make sure you're in a good place before diving into something big like the holidays.

My suggestion, as always, is to simply pre-think what you're going to do. As you gear up for the holidays, maybe go to a few extra recovery group meetings. Make enough time to talk with your support system, to confide in trusted friends and resources. Really think through what *can* be relaxed during the holiday season and what *can't*. Preparation is your best tool going into any situation. Leaning on your supports is a great way to enter potentially triggering or difficult environments from a place of strength and stability.

"NO, THANK YOU"

Even if we take the time to prepare ourselves, though, all of us know what it's like to show up to a holiday gathering and experience peer pressure. It's common at these meals to be asked to taste something that so-and-so made, with no understanding of what it will mean for you to do so. What's more, it's often a waste of time to try to explain your situation. So many people don't understand this addiction, and it can be much worse to go into detail, especially at larger gatherings.

This is another situation where I'm going to encourage you to get more comfortable saying, "No, thank you."* There are all kinds of polite, simple refusals you can employ when pressured to try a dessert: "It looks great! But I've gotta

---

* I'm a huge *Friends* fan. In one of the show's famous Thanksgiving episodes, Monica, a character who struggled with overeating from childhood into young adulthood, begins her transformation with these three simple words—"No, thank you"—after deciding enough is enough. I often think of it at family gatherings where sweets are offered to those of us in recovery.

pass." "I appreciate the sentiment, and I know you worked really hard on it." "That's not for me, but thank you." All you can do is speak the truth in love. We, of course, want to be at peace with all people, but ultimately you can't control if someone's feelings are hurt. If it's not for you, it's not for you. You will definitely end up in an uncomfortable conversation or two when you put these things into practice, but you've got to quietly do what you need to, to keep your recovery. So many times, even when people mean well, they tend to judge or criticize or share opinions that aren't helpful when you try to explain where you're coming from, or even when you don't. Get comfortable not always being understood, even by people you crave it from and love. Trust that their intentions toward you are good, and that hopefully they'll gain a better understanding down the line.

If someone is straight up bullying you, though, that's a different story. I had a client who went to a social gathering, and one of the women offered her a dessert she had made. My client politely refused and tried to pass the plate on to the next person. But the woman wouldn't let it go. When my client offered a brief but clear explanation that she couldn't have it, the woman rolled her eyes and told her to lighten up. My client ultimately left the gathering early, and when we talked about it later, we agreed that the best path out of a situation like that is to simply, graciously leave. Sometimes you've got to remove yourself from the situation if you can't find a better solution. Don't hurt *yourself* because you don't want to hurt someone's feelings.

The same goes for gifts. Oftentimes, people give sugary treats as professional gifts or as a holiday offering. It's easy to avoid them if they are gifts given to your office as a whole, but sometimes you have to deal with someone face-to-face. If I get a box of chocolates as a gift, I always thank them and say something to the effect of, "My family will enjoy this!" Whether or not you have family members to delight with a gift of chocolates, you will find a way to assert your boundaries without being rude, and in a way that lets people know that maybe this isn't the best gift for you in the future. You can always "re-gift," of course, and you are the best judge of discerning when to speak up and when to simply accept and politely dispose of someone's gift.

Ultimately, peer pressure just isn't worth it. You learned that in junior high, and you're going to learn it again in your recovery. Your boundaries are important because they keep your recovery. Your priorities are changing, because your goals are changing. Keeping your recovery is a whole different ball game than keeping your diet or keeping off ten pounds. With God's help, a good support system, and a commitment to doing what you need to do, you are going to find your way. I know it.

PART Two

PICK YOUR PATH

CHAPTER 10

Narrowing It Down

Congratulations—you've made it to Part II of our journey together! This is where we will get into the nitty-gritty of what it looks like to create a food plan uniquely suited to your needs in the recovery process. You will learn and practice the necessary skills of planning, preparation, and play. As I've said, this is not a one-size-fits-all program. But no matter how your path may look, think of this as part of your road map to freedom—mind, body, and spirit.

At this point, I hope you have a pretty clear understanding of the task before you. This book's ultimate goal is to move you toward the crafting of a food plan that is repeatable, usable, and reliable to keep you on the path of food freedom. My hope is that in reading the chapters thus far, you are feeling more empowered and enlightened as you approach what path might work best for you in this process. I hope you're starting to take to heart that you can live in a way that brings peace instead of chaos. Let's dive into a few versions this path might take.

First, take a moment to check in with yourself and take stock of where you are in the process. In light of what we've explored in Part I, where do you feel you might want to go from here? Are you feeling confident and ready to kick addictive foods to the curb? Or are you perhaps feeling anxious, aware that you need to make a change but unsure of where to start? Perhaps you're some place in between. There's no right answer to this question; we are just taking inventory before looking at some options as you begin crafting your food plan.

Maybe you're not quite ready for a food plan at all. Perhaps the concept as a whole feels overwhelming right now. That's totally OK, and it doesn't mean you have to stay in the addictive process. There are still ways to begin moving toward a food plan and making changes in your eating to get you on your way, no matter where you are. As you consider what you're ready for, remember to pray. Pray to be willing to change, for God to help you to be open and ready for healing.

PATHWAY #1: FIRST STEPS TO SATISFIED

Let me ask you another question: if you're not currently ready for a food plan, what *are* you willing to try? Perhaps you are curious about what we've been discussing and ready for a change, even if you're unsure of what that change might be. You want to take the first steps—and I want to help you take them!

If so, my recommendation for a good place to start is detoxing from added refined sugar. Cut it out completely. This is the one thing you know for certain, no matter where you're at with a food plan: sugar is addictive, and you are going to have to flush it out of your life to restore order and peace. There is no need to do this perfectly, and there is room for grace here. You also might take several attempts before it sticks, and that's OK. But a good first step of any kind toward a food plan is detoxing from sugar, so you can start the biological process of getting it out of your body's system. The next step would be to try to cut out refined white flour as well.

If you're able to accomplish those first two steps—which are no easy tasks!—and you find that you're still not ready for a food plan, then you're in good company. These "first steps" are how I started making my way toward a food plan. When I first got into recovery, as you know, I was a mess. I knew I needed help, but I certainly didn't know how to completely renovate the food in my life. At the beginning, someone encouraged me to simply try cutting out sugar first, and to stick to three meals a day with no snacking in between.

I tried and failed quite a few times at that first step before it really took. This addiction is no joke! When I finally cut sugar out for good, my eating was still quite unhealthy: I was still eating white flour, and even though I committed to eating just three meals a day, my meals were still way too big. The foods themselves were often not good for me; after a lifetime of only eating large quantities of junk food and Wonder Bread sandwiches, it was a real adjustment to eat anything that wasn't addictive. I was still drinking liters of diet soda to get me through the day, and my meals were often salads big enough for two people or a huge hoagie from Wawa. But I was starting. It was the beginning of ending my bingeing on junk food and figuring out where to begin in putting real, healthy food on my food plan.

And, to be clear, even though this was imperfect and unhealthy and I was still eating way too much food, I *was* making progress. It was a good place to start. Dialing down to just three meals a day was huge for me, and it was where I had to begin, plain and simple. Sure, I was still drinking diet soda, but I *was* learning how to get off junk food. I share this to let you know that as long as you are willing to start somewhere, even if that place feels only marginally better than where you've been, that is totally fine. Few people can quit addictive foods cold turkey and just jump into a healthier lifestyle—but change is possible with patient persistence and God on your side. All that's required to begin eating well is a willing heart.

In recovery circles, this approach is called "harm reduction."* Sometimes, even to begin breaking the cycle of addiction, you have to aim for reducing harm, and this happens by making the changes that are possible at the time. Maybe for you, that looks a bit like my first steps. Or it could mean simply being willing to try vegetables. You could start adding healthy foods into your daily food intake as you begin weaning yourself off addictive ones and recalibrating your reward system. As you develop a taste for some healthy options, you might be surprised that you enjoy how healthy food tastes. There may be certain whole foods you've never actually tried, or had prepared correctly or in a delicious way.

For instance, consider my banana muffins recipe (which you can find in the included recipe section) or try grilling vegetables with garlic—both healthy options to add to your repertoire. You can begin to change your cravings by simply showing your body that other food options are available besides cookies and chips. Once you do, the rest of the food planning begins to seem less daunting as you realize what options are available. It's all about introducing these healthier foods to your palate, step-by-step.

Even if you dread cooking, that doesn't rule out this type of path (though we encourage you to at least try your hand

---

* You can learn more about harm reduction in recovery of all kinds at www.samhsa.gov.

at cooking before you knock it altogether!). All kinds of meal delivery services exist that offer healthier, pre-made whole food options. In my practice, I've found that preparing food was sometimes the thing getting in many clients' way. Sure, they were addicted to highly processed foods, but the habit really keeping them in addiction was how much faster and more readily available junk food is. Many of my clients found it much easier to stay on the path when someone else prepared the food. So much of this process is just figuring out the practicalities of food preparation and what you can most easily and effectively work into your life.

I had a client who had to work this out for herself. She absolutely hated to cook, partly because she didn't have a great kitchen for cooking. Preparing meals was always a struggle. She wasn't a person who wanted to be in her kitchen, so she almost exclusively went out to eat. In her addiction, she often opted for fast food or other unhealthy options. In light of knowing this about herself, she began to investigate options that worked for her lifestyle.

For her, the shift involved finding the types of places that offer healthy foods, while also taking the time to investigate menu items that maybe she wouldn't have ordered before. You *can* go out to eat and find healthy food at a restaurant; you don't have to eat junk food. You just have to be open to investigating options and finding foods on the menu that are healthy and keep you out of addiction. I loved watching this client become so open to these changes. For her, letting go of highly processed foods meant embracing her own preferences surrounding cooking, and she found a path that worked for her.

Hers was a genuine transformation after she took that first baby step. And her desire for freedom grew with each next step she took toward eating well. She started at the shallow end of the pool and worked her way in, and it has proven successful. The slow, steady pace of simply being open to investigating what would work for her led to the most incredible metamorphosis. Her desire for wellness grew in tandem with her curiosity and willingness to start small.

So, where are you willing to start? There's no place too small. All it takes is the willingness to begin in order for a journey to unfold. I bet you'll be surprised how far you can get by taking one seemingly small step.

PATHWAY #2: SATISFIED WITH FIRM BOUNDARIES

This second path is for those who feel ready for a plan, and are aware that for them, structure is key. They want to take the guesswork out of food planning, and they know they're the type of person who needs specific measurements and clear, unchanging guidelines around what they eat. In most food recovery treatment circles, this is the recommended food path. As stated earlier, I differ from my colleagues in that I think there's a way to have a food plan with structure that isn't completely inflexible, but we'll get into that in the third path, toward the end of the chapter.

In this path's plan, there is absolutely no sugar, no flour, and no sugar or flour substitutes. You remove any and all foods that are potentially addictive. This food plan calls for an "all-in" mentality, where you don't take any chances. The rule of thumb is that if a food *could* be addictive, it has no place in your food plan. The idea is that you already know what foods you find addictive, and it's just not worth the trouble of even remotely investigating sugar or flour substitutes, because of the risk of being thrown back into addiction.

If this is the food plan for you, you are likely a person who needs clear structure and rules. You need to know exactly what and how much of certain foods you can eat, and have defined timelines of your meals during the day. Everything is precise—you know exactly what you're eating in exactly what amounts at exactly what time. If you have snacks in this food plan, they don't vary in type or schedule. In my opinion, you will know pretty early on if this is the food path you require, based on the self-inventory we've been doing in this book.

The motivation behind this type of food plan is to take out the guesswork that might derail you. That is, if you know exactly how much food you're going to eat, and that it's the right portion and size, there's no danger of overeating it. Where there was once only chaos around food, this plan mitigates any questions about how much is too much; if the answer never changes, then you always know the answer. If your addiction involves food-volume issues, this food plan can be hugely helpful, at least at the start of your recovery journey.

I have treated several people who found this structure and inflexibility to be a source of great clarity and peace. If this is the path that brings you peace, I recommend it wholeheartedly. Embrace the stability that taking out the guesswork brings.

PATHWAY #3: SATISFIED WITH BREATHABLE BOUNDARIES

This third path is also for those who feel ready for a food plan but who are aren't sure how rigid or flexible that plan should be. For many of us, I do think there's room for some flexibility in crafting a food plan, because life can be unpredictable.

When I was first starting out and figuring out my food plan, the rigidity of hard-and-fast structured plans felt like a straitjacket. I was told you had to weigh and measure every morsel that goes into your mouth. To be clear, I don't think that's necessarily the wrong approach. For some people, it really is what's required to keep their recovery. But I knew early on that meticulousness wasn't going to work for me. In fact, for me personally, it was just trading in one type of crazy for another. I needed to know the rules, but I needed to know how to bend them into something that worked for my life and my strengths. It's important to answer this question for yourself: Do the instructions keep me moving toward freedom, or do they feel like a different kind of crazy-making?

Regardless of your answer, as you're figuring this stuff out, it's still important to learn how to measure and weigh food. Most of us have little to no concept or gauge of correct portion sizes. If we've never learned to use a food scale, our eyeballs are probably broken from years of constantly upping our food intake to keep up with our increasing binges.

Introducing boundaries definitely helped me learn the right size for my portions, and it was incredibly useful to see how much was the ideal amount for a variety of food types. I still use a lot of the skills I learned while I was trying a more rigid food plan. For instance, I still measure grains on occasion because I don't want to overeat them, and I know if I'm not careful they can be a temptation for me. But I don't need a food scale at a restaurant. At this point in my recovery, I know the right sizes for most food groups. I know that the basic bones of any meal are going to be a few cups of vegetables coupled with a certain amount of fats, carbs, and protein. Overall, after years of refining my food plan, I've found that a routine and a structure that is free of addictive foods and mitigates haphazard eating is what works for me. I can make my choices from a peaceful place.

NARROWING IT DOWN

I learned a lot of important truths in crafting this more flexible plan. Without strict structure, I still needed to find a way in which I wouldn't be triggered, where I wasn't worried about over- or undereating, and where I wasn't eating foods that gave me problems. For example, I know that I am addicted to ice cream and cookies, not salmon. I don't feel the need to necessarily measure my salmon portions every time I have it for dinner. I *do* know that I cannot have sugar whatsoever. I can go to a restaurant with this type of flexibility and order what I have learned over the years are healthy options; then, by looking at the portions when they arrive at the table, I can determine what's the right amount and what needs to come home with me in a take-out box.

To be abundantly clear: we aren't all the same. You might try all three of the paths detailed here and find different things you like about each. There are people who need to measure all of their food all the time. For me, and for a lot of the people I've treated, there's something to be said about eating a plate of food of the right portions and ratios without worrying about it being exact or precise—all because you know it works best for you. If you get to a place where you can trust yourself, you know you're not going to overeat the stuff that's good for you (and if you do, you don't try to compensate by under-eating later).

In a way, this more flexible third path is a bit like intuitive eating. By becoming more in tune with your body's cravings once they begin to adapt and recalibrate to healthier foods, some of this stuff might come more naturally than currently feels possible. However, if you're a food addict, I don't recommend skipping meals or waiting until you're hungry to eat, because that can too easily trigger a binge.

I think it's important to stick to a schedule (again, with some flexibility) of when you eat. Think of it like this: You put gas in your tank because your car needs gas to run. You don't wait until your tank is empty, otherwise you end up stuck on the side of the road. Not eating in a regular way is a gateway for most food addicts toward bingeing and addictive behaviors.

Which brings us to another important reminder: we all need to find our food triggers.* These triggers can take many forms: specific foods, food behaviors, emotional factors, volume eating. Regardless of what food plan you end up with, this is the most important discovery to make, as it will dictate what best keeps you on the path of recovery. It informs your food plan, because it lets you know what you absolutely must avoid at all costs, and where you can afford to have a bit more flexibility.

After discovering these food triggers, you can begin to explore which food substitutes work for you. Maybe on your food plan, you can have chickpea pasta or Ezekiel bread.

---

* You can read more about this in another book of mine: *Food Triggers*.

Maybe you can have cauliflower-crust pizza. Maybe you can enjoy your morning coffee with some stevia sprinkled in.

Within the flexibility of this Satisfied Food Plan system, I like to think of foods and food groups in categories of red lights, yellow lights, and green lights. Red lights are foods you know are out for sure; yellow lights are those foods that perhaps you're figuring out how much and what substitutes work for you; and green lights are foods you know aren't a problem and that you can enjoy. For instance, green lights are all healthy whole foods, such as proteins, fruits, veggies, and brown rice. Yellow lights are foods that some may struggle with and others may not, such as nut butters and certain cereals. They're the foods where you're trying to determine what's in and what's out. Red lights are out for sure, such as sugar and white flour. I find this tool so helpful in visualizing what you know doesn't work for you while figuring out what does and might.

To be clear, even with this more flexible third path, you need some form of structure. For instance, I think it's vital to commit to no random eating throughout the day. You need to know that you're having just three meals, perhaps with a snack or two that doesn't change once you've decided how many are appropriate for your food plan. The whole point of crafting the plan is finding out the appropriate amounts and types of food to eat so that you are nourished and satisfied. That's why it's so important to do all this investigating and experimenting; you need to make sure your meals are nourishing, because you need to be full if you're only eating at specified times.

Furthermore, you can't eat in a way that's focused on weight loss. We're done with those crash diets and unrealistic eating calculations. If you don't eat enough at breakfast, you are going to put yourself in a place where you want to binge because

---

Quick Tips with Dr. Rhona: Take Caution

If you're having trouble identifying your "yellow-light" foods, consider these questions:

- Does this food (e.g., nut butter, cereal, alternative flour, etc.) make me feel confused, anxious, or obsessive? Do my cravings increase when I eat it, or do I feel in any way out of control?
- Does this food trigger volume eating for me?
- Have I ever binged on this food?

If your answer is yes to any of these questions, it's safe to say you should plan *not* to include these foods in your food plan for now.

NARROWING IT DOWN

you're hungry later in the day. Similarly, I don't recommend any type of fasting (e.g., intermittent fasting) for food addicts. It's too risky, and more often than not it sends food addicts back into the cycle of addiction. You want to set yourself up for success. Remember: this is for the long term, to keep you healthy and free from addiction over a lifetime.

Also remember that *you are not alone* in figuring this stuff out. Take advantage of the support available to you, whether that's talking to other people in recovery for advice and encouragement, or going to a nutritionist to help you put a plan in place for proper meals with all the essential elements. If you pursue the latter, make sure your nutritionist has had training in food addiction.

This is a process, and the most important thing is that you *start* it. There's absolutely no need or expectation to do it perfectly. It takes as long as it takes, and you want to find what works best for you for the lifetime ahead.

Quick Quiz with Dr. Rhona

So, which path is the one for you? To help you answer that, consider these questions:

- Are you willing to cut out sugar? [A]
- Are you looking for a totally clean slate? [B]
- Do you thrive with structure? [C]
- Are you willing to start eating structured, scheduled meals (breakfast, lunch, dinner)? [B]
- Do you know you need to start but feel like you can only do the bare minimum? [A]
- Are you willing to start cooking (or to cook more if you already do)? [C]
- Are you willing to cut out white flour? [C]
- Do you want to take the guesswork out of what you're going to eat? [C]
- Do you thrive when you know the rules but have some wiggle room? [B]

If you answered yes to mostly [A] questions, First Steps to Satisfied is probably the best plan for you. If you answered yes to mostly [B] questions, Satisfied with

NARROWING IT DOWN

> Breathable Boundaries is for you. If you answered yes to mostly [C] questions, Satisfied with Firm Boundaries is most likely the place to start for you. Remember: You can try all three! The most important thing is to *start*.

CHAPTER 11

The Building Blocks of Nutrition

> To eat is a necessity, but to eat intelligently is an art.
> —François de la Rochefoucauld

The remaining chapters (and recipes within them) in Part II are where Dietitian Jackie comes in! Her input and experience in the nutrition field will prove invaluable as you start crafting your food plan. I know you're going to love her work as much as I do. Any personal stories from here on out are Jackie's. The recipes you'll find in Part III are from both of us.

As discussed in chapter 10, a helpful way to think about approaching your food plan is the traffic light method. As a refresher, red-light items are foods that are highly addictive, like cake, cookies, chips, and fries. (For some, this category can include even "healthy" foods, such as nuts or nut butters.) Yellow-light items are foods that are challenging for some people but not all. For example, pasta, cereal, and certain grains might be yellow-light foods for you. Or you might have medical reasons, such as allergies, to avoid certain foods. If so, eliminate them from your food plan. That said, take care not to eliminate these foods simply for weight loss, as that can backfire. Over time, you might also work closely with your support system to eat measured portions of these foods and see how it goes; they don't have to stay yellow forever! Green-light foods are healthy options that do not trigger addiction, such as vegetables, proteins, and healthy fats.

No matter how you choose to categorize foods, it's important to understand why certain foods can be troublesome for food addicts. If you're feeling overwhelmed, that's totally normal! Jackie and I are here to help you every step of the way. Before we dive into the aspects of making a food plan and how to set you up for success, let's take a look at what exactly makes up your food (and what to look for on food labels).

CARBOHYDRATES

Carbohydrates are commonly referred to as both *carbs* and *starches*. Regardless of what you call them, they are divided into

THE BUILDING BLOCKS OF NUTRITION

two main categories: *complex* and *simple*. Complex carbs are defined as long chains of carbohydrates (commonly referred to as *starches*) and are found naturally in beans and whole grains. These foods contain fiber, vitamins, and minerals. According to Harvard School of Public Health, carbohydrates that contain fiber "take longer to digest—which means they have less of an immediate impact on blood sugar, causing it to rise more slowly."[11] Refined grains like white flour and white rice are technically complex since they are longer-chain carbohydrates, but because they lack fiber, they are broken down quickly and thus spike blood sugar.

Simple carbohydrates, on the other hand, are technically any monosaccharide or disaccharide (aka, one or two glucose molecules). Most fruits fall into this category. For the scientists among us, the main differentiation between complex and simple is the length of the molecule chain in the food. The main thing you need to focus on with carbs is whether you're consuming ultra-refined foods (think cookies and white bread) that have no protein or fiber and thus spike blood sugar levels, which keep you hungry; or whole foods (think fruits and vegetables) that *do* contain nutritional benefits, like vitamins and fiber, to promote fullness.

Certain kinds of carbs are challenging for those who struggle with food addiction. This is because carbohydrates start as starches, which are ultimately broken down into sugars. These sugars have shown the ability to stimulate the same addiction centers of the brain and therefore result in overproduction of hunger signals and cravings. You may be wondering: *If this is true, why doesn't everyone have a food addiction?* Well, not everyone has the same genetic makeup; some of us can live an entire lifetime without any sort of addiction, whereas others may have a genetic predisposition and be more likely to struggle with substances, like food.

The way we categorize carbohydrates will look different for everyone. If you thrive on structure and routine (like the Satisfied with Firm Boundaries Plan in chapter 10), we recommend being cautious when selecting your carbohydrates. In our experience, many people cannot tolerate any bread, tortilla, or cracker-alternative products. They are often too triggering and can mimic the sensation of red-light foods. Others who follow a more flexible structure may find these choices to be somewhat challenging (yellow) or not at all (green). Regardless of what you decide, it is best to keep the selections to a minimum at first and focus on measuring! Start with natural carbohydrate choices such as fresh fruit, sweet potatoes, brown rice, beans, and old-fashioned rolled oats. Pair these with foods rich in protein, which, like fiber, helps control those blood sugar levels we discussed earlier.

Remember: not everyone will want to include these foods in their plan. If you are someone who has struggled with bread,

THE BUILDING BLOCKS OF NUTRITION

even the healthier Ezekiel bread may be too addicting. Take a look at the options below to get a feel for what might work for you.

Complex Carbohydrate Choices	
• Beans or legumes • Brown rice • Chickpea, bean, lentil, or brown rice pasta • Corn • Creamy brown rice • Ezekiel brand: bread, pita, English muffin, tortilla	• Nut or brown rice crackers • Oatmeal • Quinoa • Sweet potato • White corn grits • White potato

Write down a few of the above options you would like to see in your plan.

_____

_____

_____

_____

FRUIT

Fruit is a sweet and nutritious simple carbohydrate; however, some fruits are considered complex because they contain longer-chain carbohydrates. For example, an unripe banana is complex, but as it ripens it turns into a simple carbohydrate—the molecular composition changes in the ripening process.

But what exactly sets the fruit apart from bread or rice? It comes down to the sugar! Fruit is filled with a type of sugar called *fructose*. What makes fructose different from typical glucose, sucrose, maltose, and lactose is its structure. Fructose can be processed and manipulated into foods that are unhealthy, but in its naturally occurring form, it's unprocessed. We recommend pairing fruit with either a protein, vegetable, dairy, or fat source. Pairing with these foods slows the digestive process, keeping you fuller, longer. Again, this is due to the added fiber, fat, or protein content, which helps minimize blood sugar spikes—which, in turn, lowers the likelihood of triggering the addiction centers of the brain.

We recommend enjoying fruit in its most natural form. When possible, purchase locally grown or unprocessed fruit. Dried fruits, on the other hand, can be tricky. Fruit naturally contains a large amount of water. When the fruit is dried, the fructose becomes concentrated. This makes the fruit taste sweeter, which is more likely to be a trigger. We recommend starting with whole fruit in its natural state before considering adding dried fruit into your plan.

THE BUILDING BLOCKS OF NUTRITION

Types of Fruit	
• Apple • Banana • Blackberry • Blueberry • Cantaloupe • Cherry • Coconut (unsweetened) • Dragon fruit • Grape • Grapefruit • Guava • Honeydew • Kiwi • Lemon • Lime • Lychee	• Mango • Nectarine • Orange • Papaya • Passion fruit • Peach • Pear • Persimmon • Pineapple • Plum • Pomegranate • Rambutan • Raspberry • Starfruit • Strawberry • Watermelon

Write down a few of the above options you might like to see in your plan.

_____

_____

_____

_____

VEGETABLES

Like fruit, vegetables fall under the green-light category but are also categorized as carbohydrates. This is why you will see some vegetables listed under the carbohydrate section, like sweet and white potatoes. Those two, along with peas and squash, are all considered "starchy" vegetables, whereas beans and legumes, technically part of the pea family, can be considered plant proteins. These starchier vegetables contain higher amounts of carbs and fiber, which contribute to what is called a glycemic index: the value assigned to a particular food based on how it can increase blood sugar levels. This number is dependent on the type of food, amount of carbohydrates, fiber, and how it's eaten.[12]

Vegetables come in a wide range of colors, flavors, and varieties. Did you know there is such a thing as purple asparagus? Or orange cauliflower? Even though these vegetables may seem completely different from the typical varieties you have seen, they often are similar in flavor profile. One advantage to eating the same foods in various varieties is you can enhance the types of vitamins, minerals, and phytochemicals in your diet. Phytochemicals are compounds found in plants that have beneficial effects, such as cancer-fighting properties, while also making your food more colorful. Many of us get stuck in the same pattern of the foods we choose, which is fine . . . until we get tired of it. So the next time you're shopping for some vegetables, try some rainbow carrots or white eggplant!

Types of Vegetables	
• Acorn squash • Artichoke • Asparagus • Beet • Bell pepper • Broccoli • Brussels sprout • Butternut squash • Cabbage • Carrot • Cauliflower • Celery • Collard green • Corn • Cucumber • Eggplant	• Garlic • Green bean • Kale • Lettuce • Mushroom • Onion • Pea • Pumpkin • Radish • Rutabaga • Spinach • Swiss chard • Tomato • Turnip • Zucchini

Write down a few of the above options you would like to see in your plan.

_____
_____
_____
_____

DAIRY

Dairy products (or dairy substitutes) are often rich in important vitamins and minerals, such as calcium, vitamin D, potassium, and magnesium. Dairy can be considered a healthy fat or protein source, helping to keep us full. Heavy cream in your morning coffee is typically a fat, whereas Greek yogurt is a protein. If you have difficulty digesting dairy products, or simply don't like them, don't worry—there are plenty of substitute options.

Dairy Choices	
Animal Sources	*Plant-Based Substitutes*
• Butter (high fat) • Cheese (high fat, low protein) • Cottage cheese • Cow, goat, sheep milk • Cream cheese (high fat) • Evaporated milk • Greek yogurt • Kefir (fermented yogurt drink) • Lactaid milk • Powdered milk • Ricotta cheese • Sour cream • Unsweetened whipped cream • Yogurt	• Almond, cashew, macadamia, flax, soy, oat, coconut, hazelnut, rice, banana, or hemp milk • Almond or coconut yogurt • Avocado, soy, or olive oil butter • Soy cream cheese • Vegan cheese • Vegan sour cream

Write down a few of the above options you would like to see in your plan.

_____

_____

_____

PROTEIN

If you were to stop a random person on the street and ask, "What is the first food that comes to your mind when you hear the word *protein*?" most would say "meat." But protein is found in both meat *and* plants. Let's first discuss why protein is so important, especially for those with food addiction.

Proteins help with the creation and regulation of hormones, bodily functions, and energy. Increased protein consumption has been linked to satiety (or fullness) and consistent blood sugar levels. This is due to hormones produced by a part of the brain called the hypothalamus, which is responsible for regulating ghrelin (hunger) and leptin (fullness); both of those greatly affect appetite, which we discussed in chapter 2.[13] For those who have difficulty with food addiction, it is critical to consume enough protein to ensure satisfaction and fullness! Protein helps us learn how to distinguish actual hunger from emotional hunger and keeps us fuller longer. The more satisfied we are, the easier it is to differentiate actual hunger from cravings. As with carbohydrates, there are two main sources of protein: animal products and plant products. Contrary to what you may have been told, it is best to consume *both* types for a well-balanced diet.

Incorporating protein at any meal or snack will help prevent mindless, impulse eating and keep you satisfied. Some individuals may need a food plan that contains more protein than others. This could be a plan that is rich in meat, fish, eggs, and dairy, or one abundant with beans, lentils, chickpeas, nuts, and dairy alternatives. If you choose to use any processed or prepackaged protein products, it is imperative to read the ingredients list. Many protein products (such as cured meats like jerky, deli meat, sausage, and bacon) are full of sugar. This is because sugar and starch are often used for flavoring and preservation. It is best to discuss any of these products with a dietitian to ensure they are the right choice for you.

While some people can tolerate sugarless lunch meats, turkey bacon, chicken sausage, or even meat substitutes, others will not be able to. Again, everyone has different needs and preferences. Take a look at the options in the next table and start considering the foods you would like to see in your plan. We've indicated combination foods—those are a protein but also contain either carbohydrates or fats.

DIFFERENCES BETWEEN FAT AND PROTEIN SOURCES

At this point you might be thinking: *Nuts are high fat, but they're also protein, right? Bacon is considered fatty, but it's also a meat, so that counts as protein, right?* Or you might be turning over other terms you've heard, such as salmon being a "fatty fish"—does that mean it counts as a fat, or a protein, or both? These questions make sense. Nutrition is not black and white. The best way to understand whether a food is considered a fat or a protein is to take a look at the grams of fat and protein, respectively, in the food.

This can get a little tricky, because most of these foods contain *both* protein and fat. If a food has seven grams of protein or more, it is a protein. If a food has eight grams of fat or more, it is a fat. But there are exceptions, which are typically called a "high-fat protein" choice. See the examples below to help you better understand how to differentiate between these two food categories.

Protein Foods 7g+	Fat Foods 8g+
Salmon: 4 oz = **25g protein**, 14g fat (both) Chicken breast: 4 oz = **35g protein**, 5g fat Turkey Bacon: 3 slices = **12g protein, 10.9g fat** (both)	Nuts: ¼ c = 5g protein, **14g fat** Nut butter: 1 tbsp = 4g protein, **8g fat** Pork Bacon: 3 slices = **8.1g protein, 8.4g fat** (both)

Protein Choices	
• Animal Sources • Chicken • Cottage cheese and ricotta cheese • Eggs • Fish or shellfish • Lamb • Lean beef • Lean pork • Milk • Processed meats: unsweetened turkey bacon, chicken sausage, uncured lunch meat • Turkey • Veal • Venison, elk, bison • Yogurt	• Plant Sources • Beans (protein and carb) • Legumes (protein and carb) • Meat substitutes (e.g., vegan meat) • Nuts (protein and fat) • Soy/tofu

Write down a few of the protein options you would like to see in your plan.

_____

_____

_____

_____

_____

_____

FATS

Fats are also classified into two main categories: *saturated* and *unsaturated*. Saturated fat is solid at room temperature—think of the marbling in a steak or the hard white coconut oil in a jar. Unsaturated fat is liquid at room temperature—like olive, canola, or avocado oil. They also differ in their sources.

Like carbohydrates, certain foods within the fats category may be triggering: nuts, nut butters, and butter, for example. We recommend being cautious with these choices, especially in the beginning. As you're figuring out what works for you, it might be best to start by choosing unsaturated fat options, such as olive oil, and focus on portion control through measuring.

Other types of fat include trans, monounsaturated, and polyunsaturated. Trans fats are found in heavily processed foods like margarine. Monounsaturated fats are found in foods like olive oil. Polyunsaturated fats are found in foods like salmon, which is also known for being rich in omega fatty acids. This information might sound confusing at first, but it's important to have at least a basic understanding of fats and where they come from, as there are many misconceptions.

For example, a lot of food companies do not tell the truth about their products. "Reduced-fat" or "fat-free" snacks are marketed to make the consumer think these products are healthier than the traditional options, when in reality they leave a person feeling unsatisfied and craving more. Did you know that the sugar content in "low-fat" or "fat-free" products is often higher than in regular products? This is because when you remove a significant amount of fat, the flavor is not as palatable. And how do these companies make these foods flavorful? By adding more sugar or artificial sweeteners. Even if they *don't* add more sugar, the overall sugar content is still higher than a comparable option with fat, because the fat has been removed, thus technically providing more sugar in one serving.

Artificial sweeteners, which we will get to later in the chapter, are tricky. For now, take a look at some of the fat choices below.

Fat Choices
• Avocado mayonnaise
• Avocado oil
• Butter
• Canola oil
• Cheese (fat and protein)
• Corn oil
• Fatty fish/omega fatty acids (salmon, tuna, sardines, anchovies)
• Mayonnaise (Duke's Real Mayonnaise does not contain sugar.)
• Nuts (fat and protein; almonds, walnuts, cashews, peanuts, pistachios)
• Nut butter (peanut, almond, sunflower, cashew)
• Olive oil
• Processed pork products (high-fat protein; bacon, pepperoni, salami)
• Seeds (sunflower, pumpkin, sesame)
• Soybean oil

Write down a few of the above options you would like to see on your plan.

_____
_____
_____

ARTIFICIAL SWEETENERS

While they are typically positioned as healthier alternatives to sugar, artificial sweeteners or other sugar substitutes—such as Splenda, Equal (aspartame), and the ever-growing list of sugar alcohols—can be as addicting as table sugar. Just because the product is marketed as a sugar alternative does not necessarily mean it should be included in your food plan. For some of us who struggle with food addiction, these products can trigger a similar reaction as table sugar. Some people are able to tolerate natural sugar substitutes (such as the plant derivatives stevia or monk fruit). Yet to start off with a clean slate, we still advise not using these products in the beginning of recovery. If you do decide to have some with your coffee or tea, pay attention to whether or not this initiates cravings. It's best to stay away from anything too much like "dessert," as it's easy to fall into binges at the outset of recovery.

Take a look at the next table. Not all these items have the word *sugar* in their name, making it more difficult to detect the hidden sugar. We recommend bringing this list with you when you go grocery shopping so you can double-check the ingredients of any new or unfamiliar product.

DECODING THE NAMES OF SWEETENERS

Sugar Choices	
• Agave nectar	• Golden syrup
• Agave syrup	• Glycerol
• Barley malt	• Grape sugar
• Beet sugar	• High-fructose corn syrup
• Brown rice syrup	• Honey
• Brown sugar	• Icing sugar
• Cane sugar	• Invert sugar
• Carob sugar	• Lactitol
• Caster sugar	• Lactose
• Coconut sugar	• Malt or maltose
• Coffee sugar crystals	• Maltodextrin
• Date sugar	• Mannitol
• Demerara	• Maple syrup
• Dextrose	• Molasses (of any variety)
• Evaporated cane juice	• Muscovado
• Fructose	• Neotame
• Fruit juice	• Palm sugar
• Fruit juice concentrate	• Panela
• Glucose	• Polydextrose

THE BUILDING BLOCKS OF NUTRITION

- Polysaccharides
- Powdered sugar
- Rapadura
- Raw/turbinado sugar
- Rice syrup
- Saccharin
- Sorbitol
- Sorghum syrup
- Sucrose
- Sugar
- Treacle
- White or granulated sugar
- Xylitol

CHAPTER 12

Food Planning

By now you are well aware that a food plan is a tool we consider vitally important to help you learn proper planning, portion control, cooking skills, and more. As you develop and begin to implement your plan, you will learn the importance of weighing and measuring, label reading, grocery shopping, meal prepping, and how to select delicious whole foods that will keep you satisfied and on track. One of the greatest things about this program is that *you* get to choose the type of food plan you want. If you can't imagine it working in your world, it probably won't. We want to teach you the skills that will become a long-term lifestyle, not just a short-term fix. Remember, this isn't punishment or another diet! It is a transformation that will keep you out of the addictive process and in freedom.

MEASURING

You may have followed diets that required you to use a point system or count calories. We do things a little differently around here. We focus on satisfaction and eating well. To start that process, we recommend that you stick to a structured plan in the beginning while you are learning appropriate portion sizes, and we highly recommend weighing or measuring your food.

If you choose to weigh your food, you will need a food scale, which is readily available through online and in-person retail stores. Be sure to place the scale on a flat clean surface, such as your kitchen counter. Press the *on* button and place a piece of parchment paper, kitchen plate, or empty container on top of the scale. Hit the *tare* button in order to "zero out" the weight of the paper, plate, or container. Add the food item. Voilà!

If you choose to measure rather than weigh your food with a food scale, we recommend using measuring cups. It's important to measure the correct foods in the correct cup, as the amounts will differ between solid and liquid ingredients. Please do not trust yourself to eyeball the ingredients in the beginning. (An exception is eating a single piece of fruit rather than exactly six ounces.) When measuring solids in a dry measuring cup—such as chopped fruit or nuts—start by overfilling the cup. Next, using the non-sharp edge of a butter knife, keep it flush with the top of the cup, and sweep it across the top, creating a level surface. This allows any excess food from the overfilled cup to return back into its original container while providing you the perfect amount of food. If you are using a wet measuring cup for liquids, such as milk, leave the measuring cup on a flat surface and get eye level with the line to ensure the measurement is correct.

While this is convenient at home, it can be a challenge to know how much you are eating when dining out. You could always ask the server to ask the chef for the portion size of each item. If you don't feel comfortable doing that, you could bring a small food scale and repeat the steps above. Or if the portion is obviously significantly more than you need, request a take-home box ahead of time and box up all of the food beyond your correct portion size. By packing up the extra food as soon as it arrives, you have your meal ready for another day and are not tempted to keep eating more as conversation lingers.

Take a look at the next tables for the correct measurement conversions for solid and liquid ingredients. You will notice spoon measurements (rather than cup measurements) included for things like nuts, nut butter, butter, oils, etc.

MEASUREMENT CONVERSIONS

Solid:

Teaspoon	Tablespoon	Cups	Ounces	Grams*
⅛ = 1 pinch				
3 tsp	1 tbsp		½ oz	14.3 g
	2 tbsp	⅛ c	1 oz	28.3 g
	4 tbsp	¼ c	2 oz	56.8 g
	8 tbsp	½ c	4 oz	113.4 g
	16 tbsp	1 c	8 oz	128 g

Depending on food type and density, gram weight conversions may vary.

Liquid:

Fluid Ounces	Cups	Pint, Quart, Gallon
1 fl oz	⅛ c	
2 fl oz	¼ c	
4 fl oz	½ c	
8 fl oz	1 c	
16 fl oz	2 c	1 pint
32 fl oz	4 c	1 quart

COOKING

You can use a variety of cooking methods as part of your food plan: steaming, blanching, braising, and grilling, to name a few. The majority of us are looking for a quick and easy way to cook our food that makes it taste great.

You may have memories as a child of your family serving canned or boiled spinach. If so, I'm sure you remember the bland, waterlogged, lifeless pile of green on your plate. Maybe you dislike spinach to this day because of it. But have you ever tried fresh baby spinach sautéed in extra virgin olive oil with minced garlic? Or what about oven-roasted asparagus with caramelized balsamic vinaigrette? Even if you're not much of a vegetable lover, you might be surprised to learn that the way we cook our food really does matter. Dried-out proteins, mushy starches, and lifeless vegetables are enough to turn anyone off! This is why it's so critical to understand how cooking affects satiety.

One of the easiest ways to cook efficiently is through meal prep or batch cooking. Even if you're not much of a chef, there are simple and easy ways to prepare a week's worth of delicious lunch and dinner options. You can do all this in under an hour! Grab your slow cooker and baking pans and get ready—but first, we're going shopping.

GROCERY SHOPPING

Have you ever experienced grocery shopping–related anxiety? Many of my own clients express this fear. They sometimes feel overwhelmed by not knowing where things are located, combined with the temptation of foods not on their plan.

Dr. Rhona also agrees that grocery story anxiety is a real thing! In addition to reacting to crowds, choices, lights, and overall stimulation, those who are overweight sometimes fear that people are judging what they are buying, according to the founder of the Binge Eating Disorder Association.[14] Whether you're a seasoned shopper or just starting out, use these tips to help equip and prepare yourself.

SHOPPING TIPS

- Always go to the store with a list, and only deviate from it for items that fit with your plan.
- Go shopping *after* a meal. Arriving at the store hungry often leads to a higher grocery bill and deviation from your plan.
- If you don't feel comfortable going into the grocery store yet—so many temptations!—experiment with Instacart or an online shopping app with curbside pickup or home delivery.

- Bring a supportive friend or spouse to help keep you on track. Or "bring" them by phone.
- Try to fill your cart with mostly fruits and vegetables; this increases the overall nutrition of your plan and decreases cost.

FOOD LABELS

While grocery shopping, find the Nutrition Facts label on the back of any food package. The nutrients are listed on a small table, typically right above the ingredients. Take a look, specifically focusing on portion size, fiber, and protein. It's best to consume products that are rich in fiber and protein because they're great for our health and help us stay satisfied. If a product has three grams of fiber or more, it is a good choice. With five grams or more, it is an excellent choice. (Be aware, though, of highly processed foods that add fiber to trick consumers—such as inulin, or chicory root fiber—always check the ingredients list! The safest fibers are raw, whole foods.) Similarly, if a product has five grams of protein or more, it is a good choice; ten grams of protein or more means it is likely an excellent choice. Again, this is because these amounts help keep us satisfied. But remember: always check the ingredients to ensure whether or not a food is in your plan.

Another important section to note is serving size. Packages list the amount of calories (along with protein, carbs, fat, etc.) per serving. Take a look at the following sample label, where a serving size is one cup, which is 280 calories. If we look more closely, we see four servings in total. So consuming the entire package would mean eating 1,120 calories, not 280—not immediately recognizable if you don't know what to look for!

SAMPLE NUTRITIONAL LABEL

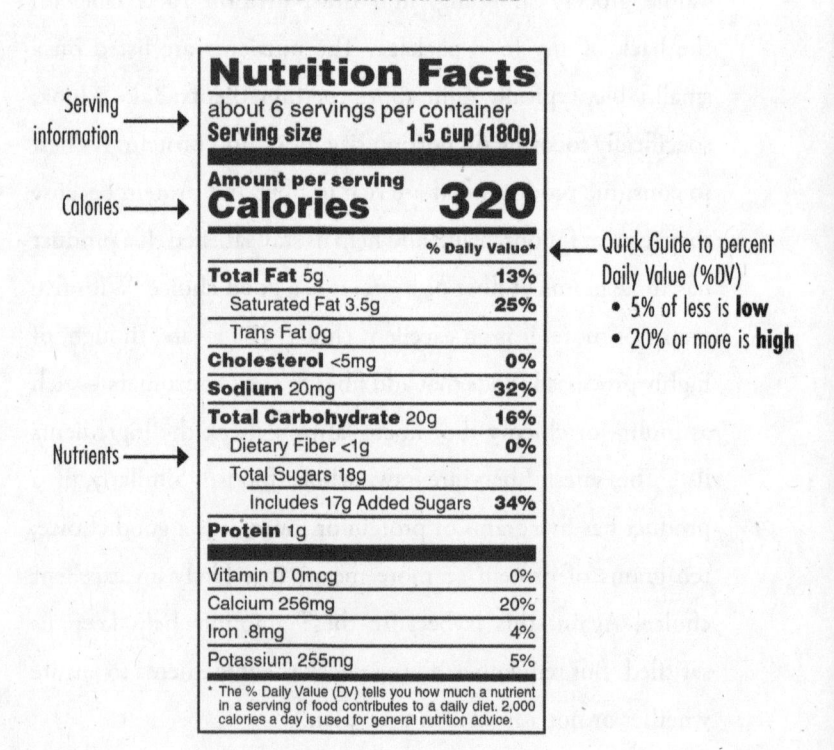

Nutrition Facts

about 6 servings per container
Serving size — 1.5 cup (180g)

Serving information

Amount per serving
Calories — 320

Calories

	% Daily Value*
Total Fat 5g	13%
Saturated Fat 3.5g	25%
Trans Fat 0g	
Cholesterol <5mg	0%
Sodium 20mg	32%
Total Carbohydrate 20g	16%
Dietary Fiber <1g	0%
Total Sugars 18g	
Includes 17g Added Sugars	34%
Protein 1g	
Vitamin D 0mcg	0%
Calcium 256mg	20%
Iron .8mg	4%
Potassium 255mg	5%

Nutrients

* The % Daily Value (DV) tells you how much a nutrient in a serving of food contributes to a daily diet. 2,000 calories a day is used for general nutrition advice.

Quick Guide to percent Daily Value (%DV)
- 5% of less is **low**
- 20% or more is **high**

The final step is to look at the ingredients list. The first five ingredients listed make up the majority of the product. If sugar or flour is listed in the first few ingredients, this is likely a highly processed product and best to avoid. However, it's still important to read the entire list of ingredients, as trigger foods could be listed toward the end. Copy the "Decoding the Name of the Sweetener" list (from a few pages back) and bring it with you to the store to determine if the products you are choosing contain sugar or flour.

HOW TO BUILD A PLATE

We understand the importance of planning, shopping, cooking, and reading nutrition labels. Now let's discuss how to build a plate. I, Jackie, grew up in an Italian family that loved to eat, which really skewed my idea of proper portion size. In Italian culture, food is everything. If you're happy, mad, sad, celebrating, mourning, or even bored, what do you do? You eat. I love to share the story about how my grandmother would make meatballs the size of softballs (no exaggeration). Plentiful amounts of food, in large volume, were common in our household. This is true for many cultures (and families), making volume, portion control, and how to build a proper plate challenging for lots of us.

For those who struggle with volume issues or have never thought about measuring, it's not an easy task. I remember my first nutrition class in college, where we learned about food groups and portions. When I saw the proper portion size of an avocado according to the U.S. Department of Agriculture (USDA), I thought to myself, *That portion is pathetic.* Over the years I learned some tips on how to combat volume issues, such as drinking a large glass of water before eating, using a salad plate rather than a dinner plate, loading up on vegetables, and, most importantly, eating satisfying, real food.

Perhaps you can relate to my stories, or perhaps volume was never your issue. Regardless, I would like you to close your eyes and picture a dinner plate in front of you. It doesn't matter if it's paper, plastic, or glass. Next, imagine a long line drawn directly down the center of the plate, creating two halves. On the right half, imagine the plate filled with delicious and flavorful vegetables, such as salad greens or roasted broccoli. Now imagine the other half of the plate being divided into fifths. These sections are filled with protein, fruit, healthy fat, and dairy. This is a representation of what your plate should contain in an ideal world. Remember, the specifics will look different for everyone; this is just an example to help you as you relearn portion sizes. Take a look at this sample image to get a better understanding:

FOOD PLANNING

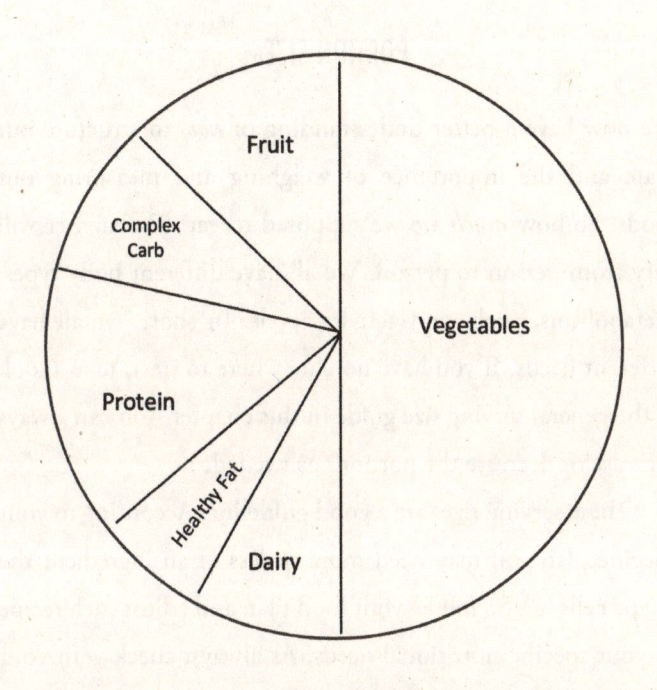

Pie chart divided into sections labeled: Fruit, Complex Carb, Protein, Healthy Fat, Dairy, Vegetables (half the chart).

Now envision how you typically build your plate. Does it look similar or different? Take notes below.

_____
_____
_____
_____
_____
_____

PORTION SIZE

We now have a better understanding of *how* to structure our plate and the importance of weighing and measuring our foods. So how *much* are we supposed to eat? The answer will vary from person to person. We all have different body types, metabolisms, goals, and activity levels. In short, we all have different needs. If you have no clue where to start, take a look at the general serving size guide in this chapter. You can always increase or decrease the portions as needed.

These serving sizes are a good guideline. According to your specific plan you may need more or less of an ingredient the recipe calls for. So follow your food plan and adjust each recipe to your specific nutritional needs. As always, check with your doctor and/or dietitian to ensure your nutritional needs are being met. If you think the Satisfied with Breathable Boundaries path is more your style and you choose to eyeball the serving sizes, follow the examples included in the guidelines:

GENERAL SERVING SIZE GUIDELINES

A special note: (**) double asterisks listed throughout this book highlight ingredients that may or may not be triggering for some individuals. Please avoid these items if you are uncertain as to how they affect you.

FOOD PLANNING

Fruit:
6 ounces raw (*about the size of a baseball*)

Vegetables:
1 cup raw (*about the size of 2 fists*)
½ cup cooked (*about the size of 1 fist*)

Protein:
3–6 ounces lean meat or poultry (*about the size of a deck of cards*)
3–6 ounces fish or shellfish (*about the size of a checkbook*)
2 whole eggs or 4 egg whites (*about 4 tablespoons*)
3–6 ounces sausage links (*1 medium-size link or 3 small links*)
3–6 ounces meatballs (*about 4 to 6 golf balls*)
2–4 pieces of bacon (protein and high fat; turkey or pork)
½–1 cup cooked beans (protein and complex carbohydrates)
½–1 cup cooked edamame or soybeans
½–1 cup cooked lentils (protein and complex carbohydrates)
3–4 oz tofu or tempeh
3–4 oz meat substitute (vegan)

Complex Carbohydrates:
½ cup cooked brown rice
12 crackers (e.g., Mary's Gone Crackers Original)**
1 small (3 ounces) sweet or white potato (*about the size of a computer mouse*)

¼ cup dry plain rolled oats to yield ½ cup cooked

1 cup cooked quinoa

½ cup cooked farro

½ cup cooked amaranth

1 cup cooked millet

½ cup cooked teff

½ cup cooked barley

1 cup cooked buckwheat

½ cup cooked sorghum

1 cup cooked spelt

¾ cup cooked freekeh

1 cup cooked kamut

Potentially Triggering Complex Carbohydrates:

Made with sprouted grains, Ezekiel bread is a healthier option than traditional white bread and can be found in several flavors.

1 slice of Ezekiel bread**

½ Ezekiel English muffin**

½ Ezekiel pita pocket**

1 Ezekiel tortilla**

½ Ezekiel hamburger bun**

½ Ezekiel hot dog bun**

2 Ezekiel hard taco shells**

2 Ezekiel waffles**

1 cup Ezekiel cereal**

1 (10-inch) corn or almond flour tortilla**
½–1 cup cooked chickpea, black bean, or rice pasta**
1 cup cooked rye**

Dairy:

1 cup milk

¾ cup yogurt

½ cup cottage cheese

1–1.5 ounces cheese *(about the size of 3 to 4 dice)* (protein and high fat; can be used as a fat)

1 tablespoon cream cheese or sour cream *(about half the size of a ping pong ball)*

1 tablespoon heavy cream *(about half the size of a ping pong ball)*

Fats:

2 tablespoons nut butter (peanut, almond, cashew, sunflower)** *(about the size of a ping pong ball)*

1 tablespoon butter, oil, or ghee *(about half the size of a ping pong ball)*

¼ cup nuts** *(about the size of a golf ball)*

¼ cup of seeds** *(about the size of a golf ball)*

⅓ avocado

Condiments:

2 tablespoons *(about the size of a ping pong ball)*

THE SATISFIED GUIDE TO EATING WELL

Sweetener-Free Condiments/Seasonings
1 tablespoon citrus juice (lemon, lime, orange, grapefruit, etc.)
Herbs (basil, dill, parsley, cilantro, etc.)
Spices (garlic powder, cumin, cinnamon, paprika, etc.)
1 tablespoon horseradish sauce
1 tablespoon yellow or Dijon mustard
1 tablespoon dill pickle spears
1 tablespoon vinegar
1 tablespoon low-sodium soy sauce or liquid aminos
1 tablespoon hot sauce
1 tablespoon plain yogurt
1 tablespoon ketchup (no sugar added option, such as Primal Kitchen)
1 tablespoon BBQ sauce (no sugar added)
1 tablespoon unsweetened salsa
1 tablespoon pesto (good fat source)
1 tablespoon salad dressing
Most condiments have hidden sugars and flour that act to flavor, preserve, and thicken. It is best to stick to condiments listed in the chart above as safe choices. Remember: always double check the ingredient list to ensure each individual product is sugar- and/or flour-free.

FOOD PLANNING

Quick Tips with Dr. Rhona: Food Plan Basics

1. Routine is key.
2. Keep it simple.
3. Make a plan and stick to it as much as possible.
4. If you're unsure, ask for support.
5. Never restrict.
6. Don't make excuses for eating addictive foods—think of it as an allergy.
7. If you get off track, start over; don't try to fix one mess by making another.
8. Always be kind to yourself, no matter how much you struggle.
9. Feed your soul every day.
10. One day at a time.

CHAPTER 13

Food Plan Examples

Armed with all this information, it's now time to begin thinking about picking your path and building your plan. Our goal is to help you achieve freedom from addictive eating and find true peace. No matter where you are currently, we want you to make steps in the *right* direction.

In light of the valuable food information we've covered so far in Part II, here are some examples of what your food plan might look like, based on your needs for either a First Steps to Satisfied pathway, a Satisfied with Breathable Boundaries pathway, or a Satisfied with Firm Boundaries pathway. Look at the options that follow and choose the path you think best suits your lifestyle. Don't be afraid to try more than one! That's what they're here for.

Each of these plans is focused on well-balanced eating with a variety of snack options. If after looking them over you find yourself desiring more options, refer to the included Appendix at the back of this book for four more plans, especially if you lead a more active lifestyle.

If you pick a plan that incorporates snacks, it's important to maintain consistency: consume your snacks at the same time each day to form steady habits, rather than grazing haphazardly or skipping your snack if you don't feel hungry. In the beginning, it may be easier to eat the same snack until the habit is formed. This could be six ounces of fruit with a hard-boiled egg, a cheese stick, or yogurt.

Remember, your plan may change over time. At first, just focus on finding the balance to feel satiated. Choose the plan that is most conducive to your current lifestyle.

FOOD PLAN EXAMPLES

Plan A

PLAN

Breakfast:
Carbohydrate: 3 oz
Fruit: 6 oz
Healthy fat: 1 tbsp or 0.5 oz
Dairy: 1 c or 8 oz

Lunch:
Protein: 3 oz Women, 4 oz Men
Fruit: 6 oz
Vegetable: 2–3 c raw or
1–2 c cooked
Healthy fat: 1 tbsp or 0.5 oz

Dinner:
Protein: 3 oz Women, 4 oz Men
Carbohydrate: 3 oz
Vegetable: 2–3 c raw or
1–2 c cooked
Fat: 1 tbsp or 0.5 oz

SAMPLE

Almond Blueberry Cereal:
**Ezekiel cereal: 1 oz
Fresh blueberries: 6 oz
**Slivered almonds: 1 tbsp or 0.5 oz
Milk: 1 c or 8 oz

Grilled Chicken Salad w/ Apple:
Sliced Chicken: 3 oz Women,
4 oz Men
Diced Apple: 6 oz
Salad greens: 2–3 c raw or
1–2 c cooked
Dressing: 1 tbsp or 0.5 oz

Salmon Sweet Potato Bowl:
Baked salmon: 3 oz Women,
4 oz Men
Sweet potato: 3 oz
Broccoli: 1–2 c cooked
Olive oil: 1 tbsp or 0.5 oz

Plan A is perfect for those who are looking to avoid snacking. You will get everything you need each day, leaving you full and satisfied. This is one of Dr. Rhona's personal favorites!

Plan B

PLAN

Breakfast:
Carbohydrate: 1 oz or ½ c cooked
Dairy: 1 c or 8 oz
Fruit: 6 oz
Healthy fat: 1 tbsp or 0.5 oz

Snack:
Protein: 2 oz
Fruit: 6 oz

Lunch:
Protein: 3 oz Women, 4 oz Men
Vegetable: 2–3 c raw or
1–2 c cooked
Healthy Fat: 1 tbsp or 0.5 oz

Dinner:
Protein: 3 oz Women, 4 oz Men
Carbohydrate: ½–1 c
Vegetable: 2–3 c raw or
1–2 c cooked
Fat: 1 tbsp or 0.5 oz

SAMPLE

Oatmeal:
Cooked oatmeal: ½ c
Milk: 1 c or 8 oz
Banana: 6 oz
**Walnuts: 1 tbsp or 0.5 oz

Eggs & Fruit:
Hard-boiled egg: 2 eggs
Grapes: 6 oz

Tuna Salad w/ Veggie Sticks:
Canned tuna: 3 oz Women,
4 oz Men
Celery & carrot sticks: 2–3 c raw
Duke's mayo: 1 tbsp or 0.5 oz

Chicken Stir-Fry w/ Rice:
Chicken: 3 oz Women, 4 oz Men
Brown rice: ½–1 c
Asian-style veggies: 1–2 c cooked
Sesame oil: 1 tbsp or 0.5 oz

Plan B incorporates the balance of Plan A with the added pick-me-up of a snack. This plan is perfect for those who need a small midmorning boost. This can be especially helpful for early risers who get hungry prior to lunchtime.

FOOD PLAN EXAMPLES

Plan C

PLAN

Breakfast:
Fruit: 6 oz
Carbohydrate: 1 oz
Protein: 2 oz Women, 3 oz Men
Healthy fat: 1 tbsp or 0.5 oz

Snack:
Dairy: 1 c or 8 oz
Fruit: 6 oz

Lunch:
Protein: 3 oz Women, 4 oz Men
Healthy fat: 1 tbsp or 0.5 oz
Vegetable: 2–3 c raw or 1–2 c cooked

Snack:
Protein: 1 oz
Fruit: 6 oz

Dinner:
Protein: 3 oz Women, 4 oz Men
Carbohydrate: ½–1 c
Vegetable: 1 c or 8 oz
Healthy fat: 1 tbsp or 0.5 oz

SAMPLE

Basic Breakfast:
Raspberries: 6 oz
**Ezekiel bread: 1 oz
Eggs: 2–3 eggs
Butter: 1 tbsp or 0.5 oz

Fruit & Yogurt:
Yogurt: 1 c or 8 oz
Strawberries: 6 oz

Chicken & Broccoli:
Chicken: 3 oz Women, 4 oz Men
Olive oil: 1 tbsp or 0.5 oz
Broccoli: 1–2 c cooked

Cheese & Fruit:
Cheese stick: 1 oz
Strawberries: 6 oz

Taco Bowl:
Lean ground beef: 3 oz Women, 4 oz Men
Cooked quinoa: ½–1 c
Roasted vegetables: 1 c or 8 oz
Olive oil: 1 tbsp or 0.5 oz

Plan C is a step up from Plan B: three meals with two snacks for those who are used to eating more frequently.

Plan D

PLAN

Breakfast:
Protein: 2 oz Women, 3 oz Men
Healthy fat: 2 tbsp or 1 oz
Fruit: 6 oz

Snack:
Dairy: 1 c or 8 oz
Fruit: 6 oz

Lunch
Protein: 3 oz Women, 4 oz Men
Vegetable: 2–3 c raw or 1–2 c cooked
Healthy Fat: 1 tbsp or 0.5 oz

Snack:
Healthy fat: 1 tbsp or 0.5 oz
Vegetable: ½–1 c raw or 1–2 c cooked

Dinner:
Protein: 3 oz women, 4 oz Men
Carbohydrate: 3 oz
Vegetable: 2–3 c raw or 1–2 c cooked
Fat: 1 tbsp or 1 oz

Snack:
Protein: 1 oz
Fruit: 6 oz

SAMPLE

Avocado, Eggs, & Fruit:
Eggs: 2–3 eggs
Avocado: 1 tbsp or 1 oz
Strawberries: 6 oz

Yogurt & Fruit:
Yogurt: 1 c or 8 oz
Blueberries: 6 oz

Chicken & Veggies:
Chicken: 3 oz Women, 4 oz Men
Roasted veggies: 1–2 c cooked
Olive oil: 1 tbsp or 0.5 oz

Cucumber w/ Dip:
**Herbed tahini: 1 tbsp or 0.5 oz
Cucumber slices: ½–1 c raw

Pork, Potato, & Veggies:
Pork: 3 oz Women, 4 oz Men
Potato: 3 oz
Broccoli: 1–2 c cooked
Butter: 1 tbsp or 1 oz

Nighttime Snack:
Cheese stick: 1 oz
Apple: 6 oz

For those who have difficulty with blood sugar dips, this plan is for you: three meals per day with three additional snacks. Consistent, healthy meals or snacks will keep you satisfied and alert all day long.

FOOD PLAN EXAMPLES

Dr. Rhona and I feel strongly about your food plan being both satisfying and nourishing. The previous options are just a few ways to keep your food delicious and exciting, all while keeping you free from addiction. That said, if you hate your plan, it's not likely to work. Don't be afraid to try more than one while you're figuring out what works best for your satiety and taste needs. That's why there's a little wiggle room baked into these plans. We want you to enjoy your food without worrying about getting it "perfect."

A NOTE ON ARTIFICIAL SUGARS

As we have mentioned before, some people are extremely triggered by artificial sugars, such as stevia and monk fruit. These are naturally occurring sugars, derived from plants.[15] Even so, for some people, use of these sweeteners reignites the addictive process. For others, they aren't an issue and are totally usable.

Date syrup or paste is another popular option that falls into this category, which is used in a handful of the recipes listed in Part III. These products simply consist of dates and water, and they tend to be less addictive because they're a fruit derivative. According to research conducted by Dr. Hyder Osman Mirghani of the Department of Internal Medicine at the University of Tabuk in Saudi Arabia, tested blood glucose levels after consumption among diabetic and non-diabetic subjects. The results found a low glycemic index (blood sugar spike) among diabetic and nondiabetic subjects.[16] In other words, dates do not cause as much of a rise in blood sugar as some other sweet-tasting products. Because of this, date syrup may be used as a replacement in some recipes where other sweeteners (such as maple syrup or honey) are typically used.

At the beginning, while you're figuring out your limits and needs, we highly recommend avoiding these products until you are certain of your reaction. We have included them in this book because for some people, they're not a problem. To be clear, we are not *recommending* that you use these products. As always, please be sure to read all the ingredients on any packaged product and talk with your support team to ensure the right decision for you. In the Recipes section, these products have been marked with two asterisks (**) to denote the possibility of triggers.

FOOD SWAP TABLE

We've given you only the bare bones of a food plan up to this point. So now you get the freedom to plug-and-play—to create what most interests you and meets your needs. Look at your food plan, then consider the interchangeable items in the table that follows. Choose different items each day to include, to chase away boredom in your eating!

A word about Ezekiel bread products: Dr. Rhona and I heartily recommend Ezekiel bread because it's not highly processed food. Rather, it's what we call "real food": no refined flour or sugar, no preservatives. Made from sprouted whole grains and legumes. That makes for a nutrient-dense part of your diet that won't increase your blood sugar.

MEASUREMENT CONFUSION

There are many schools of thought on measuring. You must understand measurements as you relearn proper portion amounts. That said, we feel passionately about ensuring you are satisfied throughout this experience. We want you to feel content with your food, so there is no *over-* or *under*eating. We recommend you try the portions we suggest, but please know they can always be adjusted based on your hunger levels as you learn what you need.

Remember to always refer to your specific plan for your specific needs. These measurements are based on general serving sizes. However, your plan may provide more than one serving size. Once again, potentially triggering foods above have been notated with a double asterisk (**).

Food Swap Table

Carb	Protein	Fat	Fruit	Veg	Dairy
½ c or 4 oz sweet potato	**Animal proteins:**	1 tbsp olive oil	1 medium apple	**Cooked vegetables:**	**1 c or 8 oz** milk
1 oz or ½ c cooked brown rice	1 oz boneless, skinless chicken breast	1 tbsp avocado oil	1 small to medium banana or ½ large	½ c or 4 oz broccoli	goat milk
1 oz or ½ c cooked quinoa	1 oz boneless skinless turkey breast	1 tbsp canola oil	1 medium orange or 2 small	½ c or 4 oz carrots	unsweetened almond milk
1 oz or ½ c cooked oatmeal	1 oz pork tenderloin or lean pork chop	1 tbsp coconut oil	1 kiwi	½ c or 4 oz spinach	unsweetened cashew milk
1 oz or ½ c cooked millet	1 oz lean beef	1 tbsp butter	1 medium peach	½ c or 4 oz kale	unsweetened coconut milk
1 oz or ½ c cooked amaranth	1 oz lamb	1 tbsp margarine	1 medium nectarine	½ c or 4 oz cabbage	unsweetened soy milk
1 oz or ½ c cooked teff	1 oz venison	⅓ avocado	1 medium plum	½ c or 4 oz cauliflower	unsweetened plain yogurt
½ c or 4 oz white potato	1 oz bison	1 tbsp heavy cream	1 medium pear	½ c or 4 oz celery	plain Greek yogurt
1 oz pasta substitute**	1 oz duck	1 oz olives	6 oz unsweetened apple sauce	½ c or 4 oz celeriac	cottage cheese
1 slice of Ezekiel bread**	1 oz turkey or pork bacon	2 tbsp guacamole	6 oz blueberries	½ c or 4 oz eggplant	¾–1 c kefir
	1 oz turkey or chicken sausage	2 tbsp hummus	6 oz strawberries	½ c or 4oz peppers	dairy-free yogurt
	1 medium to large link of sausage (any)	1 tbsp mayonnaise	6 oz raspberries	½ c or 4 oz onion	1 oz cheese
		1 tbsp unsweetened peanut butter**	6 oz watermelon	½ c or 4 oz zucchini	
		1 tbsp unsweetened almond butter**		½ c or 4 oz mushrooms	
		1 tbsp unsweetened cashew butter**		8–12 asparagus spears	

Carb	Protein	Fat	Fruit	Veg
½ Ezekiel English muffin**	1 oz shellfish	1 tbsp unsweetened sunflower seed butter**	6 oz cantaloupe	**Raw vegetables:**
½ c Ezekiel cereal**	1 whole egg	1 oz peanuts**	6 oz pineapple	1 c or 8 oz broccoli
2 Ezekiel taco shells**	3 egg whites	1 oz almonds**	6 oz fresh figs	1 c or 8 oz carrot
1 Ezekiel tortilla**	**Plant proteins:**	1 oz walnuts**	6 oz mango	1 c or 8 oz spinach
½ Ezekiel pita pocket**	1 oz tofu	1 oz pecans**	6 oz grapes	1 c or 8 oz cabbage
½ Ezekiel hamburger bun**	1 oz black beans	1 oz pistachios**	1 oz dried fruit *caution	1 c or 8 oz salad greens
1 Ezekiel waffle**	1 oz pinto beans	1 oz macadamia nuts**		1 c or 8 oz kale
1 oz Ezekiel pasta**	1 oz cannellini beans	1 oz Brazil nuts**		1 c or 8 oz spinach
	1 oz great northern beans	1 oz sunflower seeds**		1 c or 8 oz cucumber
	1 oz kidney beans	1 oz chia seeds**		1 c or 8 oz tomatoes
	1 oz garbanzo beans	1 oz pumpkin seeds**		1 c or 8 oz fennel
	1 oz lentils	1 oz flax seeds**		**Starchy vegetables:**
	1 oz veggie burger	1 oz hemp seeds**		½ c or 4 oz corn
		1 oz poppy seeds**		½ c or 4 oz parsnips
		1 oz sesame** seeds		½ c or 4 oz peas
		¼ c almond flour**		½ c or 4 oz pumpkin
				½ c or 4 oz acorn or butternut squash
				½ c or 4 oz succotash
				½ c or 4 oz rutabaga

CHAPTER 14

Commonly Asked Questions

In our work with clients and in many other interactions over the years, we have fielded a full gamut of questions related to food addiction, food planning, relearning healthy eating habits, and more. Here are our answers to some of the most frequent questions we've been asked.

What should I do about drinks like alcohol and coffee?

Overall, we recommend avoiding alcohol, because it works just like sugar in the body and is triggering. What's more, most alcoholic beverages are *full* of sugar.

Coffee is a bit different. It's definitely best to exercise caution, as so many coffee drinks (lattes, frappuccinos, mochas, et al.) can be full of sugar. If you're a latte lover, make sure you know the ingredients and insist on no sugar. Depending on the stage of your recovery, it might be possible to add stevia as a sweetener, if you can tolerate it. While we're talking coffee, this is also a good place to point out that caffeine also can be triggering because of how it's metabolized in the body. It's best to limit your intake to one to two caffeinated beverages a day, especially as you're relearning and reestablishing new patterns.

As alternatives, water and herbal tea are always great options!

Why are calories not just calories?

How is it that the calories in an apple are different from the calories in a candy bar? The answer is simple, yet complex. The simple answer is because of the contents of the food. The more complex answer has to do with energy and nutritional density. You may have heard the terms *nutrient dense* or *calorically dense*. These are often interchanged but actually have very different meanings.

Nutrient density describes foods that are high in nutrition, including fiber, complex carbohydrates, and healthy fats, as well as vitamins and minerals. Calorically dense foods are high in calories and lack nutritional value. Using the example of an apple and a candy bar, the apple is nutritionally dense, as it is rich in fiber; whereas the candy bar is calorically dense, providing little to no nutritional value but a high calorie count. However, there are healthy foods that can be both calorically and nutritionally dense, such as dried fruit. When in doubt, focus on whole, fresh ingredients.

Do I have to weigh and measure my food?

We highly encourage everyone to weigh and measure their food, at least when starting out. This way you know the exact amount you are putting into your body. It may feel like an extra step, but it allows you to accurately track your intake, which can be helpful when reporting your food plan to a recovery sponsor or dietitian. It can be a struggle to eyeball our measurements, especially in the beginning, and there's zero shame in that!

Is snacking bad?

Snacking is neither good or bad, if it's part of the food plan that works for you. If your plan calls for snacks, then they're perfectly fine. Some people, for instance, struggle with low blood sugar levels, specifically diabetics. In this scenario, having frequent small meals is OK. If you aren't sure, touch base with your food support team to help you make a decision that works for you.

Why is protein important?

Protein helps with our muscles, bones, immunity, and the creation of hormones. Protein also reduces cravings because it promotes fullness. An easy saying to remember is "protein keeps you fuller longer." It helps you stay satisfied and well-nourished, so be sure to include protein sources at each meal and snack. Protein can come from animals, plants, or both (e.g., meats, fish, eggs, dairy, beans, lentils, and soy).

As another benefit, a diet rich in protein can have positive effects on your mood. Research shows that those who regularly consume protein have higher norepinephrine and dopamine levels—that is, neurotransmitters that assist with motivation and concentration.[17] Is there such a thing as too much protein? Yes. As with any nutrient, excessive amounts can cause problems. Balance is important.

Am I not getting enough protein if I am a vegan or vegetarian?

A common misconception about vegan or vegetarian diets is that they don't provide sufficient protein without meat. It is true that animal protein products contain higher amounts of protein per serving than plant products, and plant proteins have fewer grams per serving. Yet plant products contain fiber and little to no saturated fat, unlike animal products. If you choose to follow a vegan or vegetarian diet, be sure to consult with a medical physician and/or nutrition professional to make sure it's implemented appropriately.

Why is fat important, and what are the best sources?

Believe it or not, fat can be good for us! Healthy fats are rich in vitamins A, D, E, and K. Adequate intake assists with blood sugar spikes, keeping us full and satisfied. Eating food with healthy fats helps slow down our digestion. Some examples include avocados, nuts, seeds, nut butters, and omega fatty acids from fatty fish.

Too little dietary fat has been linked with adverse mental health effects, including irritability, depression, and difficulty concentrating.[18] In studies, individuals with adequate fat intake were less likely to suffer from these effects and showed improved mental and physical health. Some of the best oils to cook with (such as avocado oil and sesame oil) are great sources of healthy fats and have the highest smoke point—meaning the oil can withstand a high heat temperature due to its composition and does not burn easily.

What about carbs; how important are they?

Despite the current craze over the ketogenic diet, which promotes a significant reduction or elimination of carbohydrates, carbs are actually extremely beneficial to our bodies. They sharpen brain function, improve glucose stability, ease digestion, and help with satiety. On average, roughly 20 percent of our carbohydrate intake is used for brain function alone! This leaves 80 percent for blood glucose stability, energy for our cells, additional fiber to help with our digestion, and overall satiety.

Evidence suggests that a diet high in ultra-processed carbs, however, has been associated with abnormal blood sugar levels and, as a result, a decrease in mental health. Individuals who consume a diet full of complex carbohydrates (instead of ultra-processed carbs) have shown decreased levels of depression and reduction in inflammatory effects.[19] So the next time you hear that carbs are bad, remember that's only half the story.

Is organic really better?

The debate over organic versus nonorganic foods has been ongoing for many years. According to researchers at Southern Cross University in Australia, the increased demand for organic products has grown rapidly over the last few decades.[20] The main benefit of organically grown food is its lack of pesticidal chemical use. On the other hand, conventional growing provides a significant benefit to the extreme demands of the world's food supply chain by preventing crop-related damage and disease.

While seeing both sides, we believe that a lifestyle rich in organic fruits and vegetables is critical for those who suffer from food addiction. The vitamins, minerals, and fiber play a critical role in helping you feel satisfied and full, in addition to being low in caloric value and rich in nutrients. For some unique and flavorful ways to incorporate more of these foods in an addiction-free way, take a look at the recipes in Part III.

COMMONLY ASKED QUESTIONS

What is the deal with gluten, and why is it seen as the enemy?

In short, gluten is a protein found in many grains. The gluten-free diet has gained popularity over the years as gluten sensitivities and intolerances, along with information about celiac disease, have become more common. Unfortunately, diet culture has manipulated this as a method to lose weight. Gluten sensitivity and celiac are *not* the same. According to Northwestern Medicine, the difference between the two diagnoses lies in the immune system. Celiac disease is defined as a "genetic autoimmune disease where wheat triggers antibodies to attack the small intestine."[21] This diagnosis is determined by a blood test or biopsy. Gluten sensitivity, on the other hand, is not considered an autoimmune disorder. It's determined by a false celiac blood test, along with the elimination of other potential allergies.

Whether an individual is gluten sensitive or is diagnosed with celiac disease, specific foods should be avoided (or implemented only under the specific instruction of medical/nutritional experts). Making dietary changes without proper instruction can lead to malnourishment and severe nutrient deficiencies. If you have been diagnosed with gluten intolerance, here is a short list of foods to avoid and a few others to enjoy.

Avoid: Wheat flour, rye flour, barley flour, triticale, graham flour, bulgur flour, farro, farina, durum flour, kamut, bromated flour, spelt, wheat berries

Enjoy: Quinoa, brown rice, buckwheat flour, tapioca, arrowroot, oats (if processed in a facility that is gluten-free), wild rice, sorghum, millet, amaranth, teff, corn

I've heard conflicting advice about the importance of water. Can you help?

Absolutely! Did you know that the human body is made up of roughly 60 percent water? So it's no surprise that staying hydrated is critical to our mental and physical health. The debate over how much water to consume daily has changed over the years. According to the USDA, adults nineteen and older should consume anywhere from nine to thirteen cups of water per day (roughly 72–104 fluid ounces).[22] Check with your doctor regarding what's best for you.

Many of us struggle with water intake because we are busy, forgetful, or simply dislike water. A few hydration tips: carry a reusable water bottle, add natural flavoring to enhance the taste (fresh herbs, sliced cucumber, or lemon juice), set alarms to remind yourself to drink, and consider unsweetened beverages (mocktail, iced tea, or seltzer water) to keep hydration interesting.

COMMONLY ASKED QUESTIONS

Can I do it all with diet alone? How much does exercise matter?

When we eat a balanced diet filled with fruits, vegetables, whole grains, lean proteins, healthy fats, and dairy, our body is able to absorb all the energy it needs. That energy then helps our body function. So diet and exercise really go hand in hand.

According to experts, adults should perform at least 150 minutes of moderate-intensity exercise per week; in other words, thirty minutes a day, five days a week.[23] This can look a bit different from person to person, but the main purpose is to get moving, however that may look in *your* life. You might start by parking at the far end of the lot, doing chair exercises, or taking the stairs when given the option. Start with low intensity; you can always work your way up! But remember to clear any form of physical activity with your doctor first.

FINAL THOUGHTS

Congratulations—you've made it through Parts I and II! Take a minute to celebrate. It's no small accomplishment. Think about where you were when you started reading this book. You are now equipped with so much more information, insight, and actionable items to create lasting, freeing change in what you eat. You no longer have to be stuck in the battle of food addiction. You are one *huge* step closer to being free of the chaos and confusion of the addictive cycle. We are *so* proud of you, and so excited for the freedom awaiting you in your future. The recipes in Part III are the next step in this journey.

A reminder: you don't have to do any of this alone! Lean on your supports. Consult a dietician to work on a plan that's best for your needs. Phone someone further ahead in the recovery process, and ask for help when you need it. You've got this—with God's help.

PART Three

TRANSFORM YOUR MEALTIMES

As you cook, you'll want to focus on well-balanced foods to assist with craving reduction, satisfaction, and improved nutrition. Check out the fresh ingredients, familiar flavor profiles, and simple instructions in our recipes to follow. We've created healthy choices for every occasion: breakfast, lunch, snacks, dinner—even holiday meals. On many recipes, we've added optional ingredients so you can better tailor each dish to your taste; and we've suggested some substitutions. You know your dietary requirements best, so always tailor these recipes as needed for gluten-free, dairy-free, vegan, or vegetarian diets.

Think of these recipes as the start of a cookbook you'll be able to pull from for years to come. Happy cooking!

General Disclaimer: These recipes are estimations of nutrients and utilize the "satisfied way" of doing things. Measurement methods, food products, serving sizes, and nutrient values will vary individual by individual. The following recipes are based on the standard portion sizes shown on previous pages, but they may contain more than one portion. Please adjust to your specific needs and always refer to your support team for assistance. Should you wish to have these recipes customized to your specific plan, please schedule an appointment with your preferred nutritionist.

BREAKFAST RECIPES

Everyone's Favorite Banana Muffins

INGREDIENTS:

- 5 ripe bananas, peeled and mashed
- ½ cup unsweetened applesauce
- 3 cups rolled oats
- 1 tablespoon cinnamon
- 1 tablespoon baking powder
- 1 teaspoon vanilla extract
- 1 cup raisins

INSTRUCTIONS:

1. Preheat the oven to 350 degrees. Place 12 liners into a 12-cup standard muffin tin.
2. In a large bowl, combine the bananas and applesauce and stir with a spatula to mix well. Add the oats, cinnamon, baking powder, and vanilla and mix just until moistened. Fold in the raisins.
3. Grease the muffin pan. Fill each muffin cup fully, as these muffins do not rise. Bake for about 20 minutes, until the tops of the muffins are golden brown. Store muffins in an airtight container for up to 5 days at room temperature.

Recipe yields: 12 muffins (single serving size: 2 muffins)

Mediterranean Frittata

INGREDIENTS:

- 1 tablespoon olive oil
- 8 large eggs
- 1 cup spinach, chopped
- ¼ cup sun-dried tomatoes, chopped
- 1 small white onion, diced; or 1 small leek, white part only, diced
- ¼ teaspoon salt
- ½ teaspoon black pepper
- 3 ounces goat cheese, crumbled

INSTRUCTIONS:

1. Preheat the oven to 400 degrees. Brush a 9.5-inch pie dish with the oil and set aside.
2. Beat the eggs in a large bowl until frothy. Add the spinach, sun-dried tomatoes, onion, and salt and pepper. Mix to combine. Pour the egg mixture into the prepared baking dish. Sprinkle the goat cheese over the top of the egg mixture.
3. Bake for 25 minutes, or until the egg is set. Slice into 8 slices and serve warm.

Recipe yields: 4 servings

Greek Avocado Toast

INGREDIENTS:

- 2 large eggs
- ⅓ avocado
- 1 slice Ezekiel bread, toasted
- ½ cup baby spinach
- 2 thick tomato slices
- 1 ounce feta cheese
- Pinch of black pepper

INSTRUCTIONS:

1. Cook the eggs to desired consistency.
2. Smash the avocado onto the toast. Add the baby spinach on top of the avocado and the tomato on top of the spinach. Place the eggs on top of the tomato. Top with the feta cheese and pepper.

Recipe yields: 1 serving

Eggs in a Nest

INGREDIENTS:

- 2 large sweet potatoes, peeled and grated
- 2 tablespoons olive oil
- 1 teaspoon onion powder
- 1 teaspoon garlic powder
- 1 teaspoon salt
- ¼ teaspoon pepper
- 6 large eggs

INSTRUCTIONS:

1. Preheat the oven to 425 degrees. In a medium bowl, mix together the potatoes, oil, onion powder, garlic powder, salt, and pepper.
2. Add ⅓ cup potato mixture to 6 cups of a standard muffin pan. Using a shot glass or a spoon, press the mixture down to create a small crust or nest with the potatoes. Bake the empty nests for 15 to 25 minutes, until crisp.
3. Remove the nests from the oven. Add 1 egg into each nest. Return to the oven and bake for another 10 to 15 minutes, until the egg whites are cooked and yolks are the desired consistency.

Recipe yields: 3 servings (single serving size: 2 nests)

No Sugar Granola

INGREDIENTS:

- 8 cups old-fashioned oats
- 1 cup raisins
- ½ cup slivered almonds
- ½ cup chopped walnuts
- ½ cup sunflower seeds
- 1 cup shredded, unsweetened coconut
- ¼ cup olive oil
- ¼ cup frozen apple juice concentrate, thawed
- ¼ cup date syrup or paste**
- 1 tablespoon cinnamon

INSTRUCTIONS:

1. Preheat the oven to 350 degrees. Place all the dry ingredients on a baking sheet and bake for 7 minutes, tossing halfway through. Remove from the oven.
2. In a small bowl, combine the oil, apple juice concentrate, date syrup, and cinnamon. Stir to mix well. Pour the mixture over the dry ingredients and toss to coat. Return the granola to the oven and bake for another 7 minutes, tossing halfway through.

Enjoy this granola with yogurt, fruit, or milk.

Recipe yields: 32 servings (single serving size: ¼ cup)

Satisfied Breakfast Skillet

INGREDIENTS:

- 4 strips uncured, sugarless bacon
- 1 medium white onion, finely chopped
- 2 cups white potatoes, unpeeled and cubed
- 2 cloves garlic, minced
- ¼ cup water
- 1 teaspoon salt
- 1 teaspoon black pepper
- 1 teaspoon smoked paprika
- ½ cup cheddar cheese, shredded
- 6 eggs or 12 ounces tofu
- 2 green onions, chopped

INSTRUCTIONS:

1. Heat a large skillet over medium-high heat. Add the bacon and cook until crispy. Remove the bacon to a paper-towel-lined plate.

2. Lower the heat and sauté the onion and potatoes in the remaining bacon grease until the onions are transparent, about 4 minutes. Add the garlic and water to the skillet. Cover the skillet and cook for 5 to 10 minutes until the potatoes have softened.

3. Uncover the skillet and sprinkle the potatoes with salt, pepper, paprika, and shredded cheese. Using a spatula or spoon, make 6 spaces for the eggs or tofu. If using eggs, crack them into the open spaces and cook for about 10

minutes or until the eggs are cooked through. If using tofu, separate into 6 pieces, place in the open spaces, and cook for 10 minutes. Remove the skillet from the heat.
4. Crumble the crispy bacon over the top and finish with the green onions.

Recipe yields: 4 servings

Scrumptious Banana Oat Pancakes

INGREDIENTS:

- 1 ripe banana, peeled
- ½ cup rolled oats
- 1 egg
- Splash of milk
- 1 teaspoon baking powder
- 1 teaspoon cinnamon
- 1 teaspoon vanilla extract
- Pinch of salt
- 2 tablespoons chia seeds** (optional)
- 2 teaspoons canola oil

INSTRUCTIONS:

1. In a blender, add the banana, oats, egg, milk, baking powder, cinnamon, vanilla, and salt. Blend until smooth. Add the chia seeds to the mixture after blending (to retain their crunch).
2. Heat a large skillet over medium-high heat. Add the oil. Scoop ¼ cup batter into the skillet for each pancake. Cook and flip the pancakes until both sides are golden brown.
3. Serve with fruit and yogurt if desired.

Recipe yields: 4 small pancakes (one serving)

Healthy Breakfast Cookie

INGREDIENTS:

- 2½ cups rolled oats
- ½ cup almond flour**
- ¼ cup dried, unsweetened fruit (blueberries, cranberries, or raisins)
- 1 cup chopped walnuts**
- 1 cup unsweetened almond butter**
- 2 ripe bananas, mashed
- ½ cup unsweetened almond milk
- 1 tablespoon cinnamon
- ½ teaspoon baking powder
- 1 teaspoon baking soda
- 2 shots vanilla cream stevia**
- 2 tablespoons ground flaxseed
- 4 tablespoons unsweetened shredded coconut
- 4 tablespoons date syrup**

INSTRUCTIONS:

1. Preheat the oven to 400 degrees. Line a baking sheet with parchment paper.
2. Add all the ingredients to a large bowl and mix with a spatula to combine.
3. Form each cookie with ⅛ cup of dough mixture, place onto the baking sheet, and slightly flatten. Space the cookies about 1½ inches apart. Bake for 20 minutes or until the cookies are slightly golden in color.

RECIPES

4. Remove the cookies from the baking sheet and allow to cool on a baking rack. Then transfer into an air-tight container and store in the refrigerator for up to 5 days.

Recipe yields: 12 cookies (single serving size: 2 cookies)

Mini Crustless Quiches

INGREDIENTS:

- 1 tablespoon olive oil
- 6 large eggs
- 1 cup spinach, chopped
- ½ cup bell pepper, diced
- ½ cup yellow onion, diced
- ¼ cup cheese (mozzarella, colby jack, Swiss, or muenster), grated
- ½ teaspoon salt
- ½ teaspoon pepper

INSTRUCTIONS:

1. Preheat the oven to 375 degrees. Line a 12-cup standard muffin pan. Brush the inside of the liners with the oil to help with sticking.
2. Add the eggs to a medium bowl and beat with a whisk or fork until frothy. Add the spinach, pepper, onion, cheese, salt, and pepper and mix to combine. Pour the egg mixture into the muffin cups, filling about ¾ full.
3. Bake for 20 to 25 minutes, until golden brown and the egg is set. Allow the quiche to cool slightly before removing from the pan and the liners. Enjoy warm or at room temperature. Refrigerate or freeze leftovers in a sealed container.

Recipe yields: 12 mini quiches (single serving size: 4 quiches)

Sweet Potato Crust Breakfast Pizza

INGREDIENTS:

Crust
- 2 large sweet potatoes, washed, peeled, and cut into 1-inch cubes
- 1 teaspoon salt, plus a pinch, divided
- 1 tablespoon olive oil
- 1 teaspoon pepper

Filling
- 1 teaspoon olive oil
- 1 green onion, white and green parts separated and chopped
- ½ cup bell pepper, diced
- ½ cup mushrooms, diced
- ½ cup spinach, chopped
- 2 ounces mozzarella cheese
- 4 ounces ground turkey or chicken sausage
- 5 eggs

INSTRUCTIONS:

For the crust:

1. Preheat the oven to 400 degrees.
2. In a large pot, add the sweet potatoes with enough water to just cover the potatoes, and a pinch of salt. Boil the potatoes until they are fork tender, 10 to 12 minutes. Drain the potatoes and pat them dry.

3. Add the warm sweet potatoes to a large, greased pie pan. Mash the potatoes with a potato masher or the bottom of a measuring cup and press them firmly and evenly over the bottom and up the sides of the pan to form a crust. Build the sides a bit higher, as they will shrink when baked.
4. Drizzle the crust with oil and sprinkle with salt and pepper. Bake for about 40 minutes or until firm. The crust will shrink some.

For the filling:

1. While the crust is baking, heat the oil in a skillet over medium heat. Sauté the white parts of the onion with the bell pepper and mushrooms until tender, 4 to 5 minutes. Add the turkey and brown it, another 4-5 minutes, breaking into smaller pieces. Add the spinach and cook just until it begins to wilt. Remove from the heat.
2. Remove the crust from the oven and sprinkle the cheese over the bottom of the crust. Top with the sautéed vegetables and ground turkey. Return to the oven and bake for 5 minutes, until the cheese has melted.
3. In a small bowl, whisk the eggs until frothy. Pour the eggs over the pizza and bake for an additional 5 to 10 minutes, until the eggs are cooked to liking. Allow the pizza to sit for a couple minutes to fully set. Sprinkle with reserved chopped green onion and slice.

Recipe yields: 4 servings

LUNCH RECIPES

Portobello Pizzas

INGREDIENTS:

- 2 portobello mushroom caps
- 1 tablespoon olive oil
- ½ white onion, diced
- 1 clove garlic, minced
- ⅓ cup tomato puree
- 1 tablespoon tomato paste
- ¼ teaspoon dried oregano
- ¼ teaspoon dried Italian parsley
- Pinch of salt
- Pinch of black pepper
- 1 ounce mozzarella cheese
- 4 ounces cooked chicken sausage, unsweetened

INSTRUCTIONS:

1. Preheat the oven to 350 degrees. Line a baking sheet with parchment paper.
2. Using a damp paper towel, remove any external dirt from the mushroom caps. Remove the stalks. Using a small spoon, scrape out the "gills" of the mushroom. Once cleaned, place the mushrooms gill-side down on the baking sheet and bake for 10 minutes. The mushrooms will shrink slightly and darken.

3. While the mushrooms are cooking, make the pizza sauce. Add the oil to a medium skillet over medium heat. Once the skillet is hot, add the onion and garlic and sauté until fragrant, 2 to 3 minutes. Add the tomato puree, tomato paste, oregano, and parsley. Bring the sauce to a boil, then lower the heat and simmer for 7 to 10 minutes, stirring occasionally. Season with salt and pepper.
4. Remove the mushrooms from the oven and flip them over. Spoon the sauce into the caps and top each with cheese and sausage. Return to the oven and bake for 10 minutes, until the cheese has melted and the sauce is bubbly. Serve immediately.

Recipe yields: 1 serving (2 mushroom caps)

Cauliflower Fried Rice

INGREDIENTS:

- 2 tablespoons sesame oil
- 2 cloves garlic, minced
- 1 (24-ounce) package of frozen cauliflower rice
- 1 (12-ounce) package of frozen carrots and peas
- 8 ounces mushrooms
- 10 ounces fresh spinach
- 2 tablespoons low-sodium soy sauce or liquid aminos
- 1 tablespoon onion powder
- 1 teaspoon ground ginger
- ¼ teaspoon black pepper
- Protein of your choice: 6 eggs, scrambled; or 1 block tofu, stir-fried; or 1 pound chicken, cooked
- Pinch of salt

INSTRUCTIONS:

1. Cook protein first and set aside.
2. Heat a large skillet or wok over medium heat. Add the sesame oil and garlic and cook just until the garlic is fragrant, about 1 minute.
3. Add the cauliflower rice, carrots and peas, and mushrooms to the pan. Cook until slightly tender, 5 to 7 minutes.
4. Lower the heat and add the spinach to the pan. Cook just until wilted, 1 to 2 minutes. Add the cooked protein.
5. Add the soy sauce, onion powder, ginger, salt, and pepper and stir to mix well. Remove from heat, portion, and serve immediately.

Recipe yields: 4 servings

Tasty Tuscan Vegetable Soup

INGREDIENTS:

- 2 tablespoons olive oil
- ½ large onion or 2 leeks (white parts only), diced
- 2 cloves garlic, minced
- 1 large carrot, diced
- 1 large celery stalk, diced
- 1 red bell pepper, diced
- 1 medium zucchini, diced
- 1 teaspoon dried basil
- 1 teaspoon dried oregano
- Pinch of sea salt
- Pinch of black pepper
- 4 cups vegetable broth
- 4 whole Roma tomatoes, chopped
- 1 (15-ounce) can cannellini beans, drained and rinsed

INSTRUCTIONS:

1. Heat a 4-quart pot over medium heat. Add the oil, onion, and garlic and sauté until the onion is transparent, 2 to 3 minutes. Add the carrot, celery, bell pepper, and zucchini. Cook the vegetables, stirring occasionally, for 10 minutes.
2. Season the vegetables with basil, oregano, and salt and pepper to taste. Add the vegetable stock, tomatoes, and beans to the pot. Lower the heat and simmer for 15 minutes.
3. Remove the pot from the heat and allow to cool slightly, then blend with an immersion blender until smooth.

Recipe yields: 4 total servings (single serving size: 1 cup)

Pizza Wrap

INGREDIENTS:

- 1½ cups raw vegetables (consider spinach, mushrooms, and onions), chopped
- 1 teaspoon olive oil
- 1 brown rice or sprouted grain wrap (such as Food for Life Ezekiel)**
- 2 tablespoons unsweetened tomato sauce
- 1 clove garlic, minced
- 1½ ounces mozzarella, shredded
- 2 ounces ground turkey, seasoned and cooked

INSTRUCTIONS:

1. Preheat the oven to 350 degrees.
2. Heat the oil in a medium frying pan, then brown the ground turkey, drain, and set aside. In the same skillet, sauté the veggies. Remove from the heat.
3. Line a baking sheet with parchment paper or foil. Place the wrap on the baking sheet and top with the tomato sauce and garlic. Add the cheese, vegetables, and meat.
4. Bake the pizza for about 5 minutes, until the cheese is melted and the wrap edges are browning.

Recipe yields: 1 serving

Black Bean Vegetable Soup

INGREDIENTS:

- 2 tablespoons olive oil
- 2 large carrots, peeled and diced
- 2 large stalks celery, diced
- 1 white onion, diced
- 4 cloves garlic, minced
- 2 teaspoons cumin powder
- 1 teaspoon smoked paprika
- 1 teaspoon dried oregano
- 1 teaspoon onion powder
- 1 teaspoon garlic powder
- Pinch of salt
- Pinch of black pepper
- 2 cups vegetable broth, divided
- 3 (15-ounce) cans black beans, drained and rinsed, divided

Optional toppings:

- 1 teaspoon cilantro leaves, minced
- ¼ lime, squeezed

INSTRUCTIONS:

1. Heat the oil in a large pot over medium heat. Add the carrots, celery, and onion and sauté until soft, about 10 minutes. Add and lightly sauté the minced garlic.
2. Add the cumin, smoked paprika, oregano, onion powder, garlic powder, salt, and pepper to the vegetables and cook until fragrant. Add 1 cup broth and 2 cans of black beans to the pot.

RECIPES

3. Add the remaining 1 cup of broth and 1 can of black beans to a blender. Blend until smooth. Add the pureed bean mixture to the pot and bring the soup to a boil. Lower the heat and simmer for 20 minutes, stirring occasionally. Taste and add more salt and pepper if desired.
4. Serve hot and top with cilantro and a squeeze of lime juice.

Recipe yields: 6 servings (single serving size: 1 cup)

Sweet Potato Quiche Florentine

INGREDIENTS:

- 2 large sweet potatoes, washed, peeled, and cut into 1-inch cubes
- 1 teaspoon salt, plus a pinch, divided
- 1 tablespoon olive oil
- 1 teaspoon black pepper
- 1 tablespoon butter
- 1 shallot, sliced thinly
- 1 clove garlic, minced
- 1 cup raw spinach
- 3 eggs
- 1 cup milk
- 1/3 teaspoon nutmeg, grated
- Zest of 1 lemon
- 3 ounces Swiss cheese, shredded

INSTRUCTIONS:

For the crust:

1. Preheat the oven to 400 degrees.
2. In a large pot, add the sweet potatoes with enough water to just cover the potatoes, and a pinch of salt. Boil the potatoes until they are fork tender, 10 to 12 minutes. Drain the potatoes and pat them dry.
3. Add the warm sweet potatoes to a large, greased pie pan. Mash the potatoes with a potato masher or the bottom of a measuring cup and press them firmly and evenly over the bottom and up the sides of the pan to form a crust. Build the sides a bit higher, as they will shrink when baked.

4. Drizzle the crust with oil and sprinkle with salt and pepper. Bake for about 40 minutes or until firm.
5. When the crust is ready, remove it from the oven and reduce the oven temperature to 350 degrees.

For the filling:

1. Meanwhile, in a frying pan, melt the butter. Add the shallot and garlic, cooking until softened, then add the spinach. Cook until wilted and set aside.
2. In a separate, small bowl, whisk the eggs, milk, salt, pepper, nutmeg, and lemon zest. Add the Swiss cheese and whisk well.
3. When the crust is ready, top it with the spinach mixture, then pour the egg mixture over it all.
4. Bake for 30–35 minutes at 350 degrees until settled.

Recipe yields: 3 servings

Grilled Chicken Salad with Dijon Vinaigrette

INGREDIENTS:

Dressing (enough to save some for later)
- 2 tablespoons red wine vinegar
- ½ teaspoon onion powder
- ½ teaspoon garlic powder
- 1 teaspoon Dijon mustard
- 3 tablespoons olive oil
- ⅛ teaspoon salt
- ¼ teaspoon black pepper
- ⅛ teaspoon dried oregano

Salad
- 4 ounces grilled chicken breast, sliced
- 2 cups salad greens (spinach, spring mix, or romaine)
- ¼ cup carrot, shredded
- ¼ cup cherry tomatoes
- ¼ cup cucumber, sliced
- 1 tablespoon dry roasted sunflower seeds**

INSTRUCTIONS:

1. In a small bowl or jar with a leakproof lid, combine the vinegar, onion powder, garlic powder, mustard, oil, salt, pepper, and oregano. Whisk or shake to mix well.
2. To a medium bowl, add the grilled chicken, greens, carrot, tomatoes, cucumber, and sunflower seeds. Top with 1 tablespoon vinaigrette and toss to combine.

Quick tip: this dressing makes a great everyday go-to vinaigrette for salads of all kinds!

Recipe yields: 1 serving

Asian Sesame Cashew Salad

INGREDIENTS:

Dressing
- 1 tablespoon sesame seeds**
- 2 tablespoons sesame oil
- 2 tablespoons low-sodium soy sauce or liquid aminos
- 1 clove garlic, minced
- 1 tablespoon date syrup** (optional)

Salad
- 2 cups green cabbage, shredded
- 1 cup kale, chopped (or additional shredded cabbage)
- 4 green onions, chopped
- 1 cup carrots, shredded
- 8 ounces chicken breast, cooked and shredded
- ½ cup cashews**
- 1 cup shelled edamame beans
- ⅓ cup cilantro leaves, chopped

INSTRUCTIONS:

1. In a small bowl or jar with a leakproof lid, combine the sesame seeds, sesame oil, soy sauce, garlic, and optional date syrup. Stir or shake to mix well.
2. In a large bowl, combine the cabbage, kale, green onion, and carrots. Toss to mix. Top the salad with the chicken, cashews, edamame, and cilantro. Add 2 tablespoons of dressing, then toss and serve immediately.

Recipe yields: 2 servings

Ancient Greek Salad

INGREDIENTS:

Dressing (enough to save some for later)
- 4 tablespoons olive oil
- 2 lemons
- 1 tablespoon oregano
- 2 cloves garlic, minced
- ¼ teaspoon salt
- ¼ teaspoon black pepper

Salad
- 2 heads of romaine lettuce, washed, dried, and chopped
- 1 red bell pepper, chopped
- 2 large cucumbers, sliced
- ½ cup kalamata olives, drained
- ½ large red onion, minced
- 1½ cups cherry tomatoes
- 4 ounces feta cheese
- 16 ounces cooked salmon or chicken divided into 4 servings

INSTRUCTIONS:

1. For the dressing, first zest one of the lemons for 1 tablespoon zest. Then squeeze both lemons for 4 tablespoons of juice. In a small bowl or jar with a leakproof lid, combine the oil, lemon zest, lemon juice, garlic, salt, and pepper. Whisk or shake to mix well.

RECIPES

2. In a large bowl, combine the lettuce, bell pepper, cucumbers, olives, onion, and tomatoes.
3. Right before serving, crumble the feta on top of the salad. Portion the salad and add 1 tablespoon dressing per person.

Recipe yields: 4 servings

Kale, Beet, and Goat Cheese Salad

INGREDIENTS:

Dressing (enough to save some for later)
- 1 clove garlic, minced
- 1 lemon, juiced (2 to 3 tablespoons)
- 2 tablespoons olive oil
- 1 tablespoon date syrup**
- 1 tablespoon Dijon mustard
- 2 tablespoons white wine vinegar or rice vinegar
- Pinch of sea salt
- Pinch of red pepper flakes

Salad
- 1 (15-ounce) can chickpeas, drained and rinsed
- 1 beet, peeled and chopped
- 2 tablespoons olive oil
- 1 tablespoon paprika
- 1 tablespoon garlic powder
- 1 bunch of kale, finely chopped
- ½ pound Brussels sprouts, finely chopped
- ½ cup pumpkin seeds**
- 1 cup red grapes, each cut in half
- 4 ounces soft goat cheese

INSTRUCTIONS:

1. Preheat the oven to 400 degrees and line a baking sheet with parchment paper.

2. Meanwhile, in a small bowl or jar with a leakproof lid, combine the garlic, lemon juice, oil, date syrup, mustard, vinegar, salt, and pepper flakes. Whisk or shake to mix well.
3. When the oven is heated, add the chickpeas and chopped beet to the baking sheet. Drizzle with oil and season with the paprika and garlic powder. Bake for 30 minutes.
4. In a large salad bowl, combine the chopped kale, Brussels sprouts, pumpkin seeds, grapes, and goat cheese.
5. Add the baked chickpeas and beets to the salad. Pour 4 tablespoons dressing over the salad and toss to combine.

Recipe yields: 4 total servings

DINNER RECIPES

Easy Yummy Chicken

INGREDIENTS:

- ½ cup almond flour
- 2 tablespoons parmesan cheese
- 1 teaspoon salt
- 1 teaspoon black pepper
- 1 teaspoon garlic powder
- 1 teaspoon paprika
- 1 teaspoon basil
- 1 large egg
- 1 pound chicken breast, thinly sliced, or chicken tenders
- 1 tablespoon olive oil
- 1 tablespoon butter
- 1 tablespoon minced garlic (or 6 cloves garlic, minced)

INSTRUCTIONS:

1. Add the almond flour, parmesan, salt, pepper, garlic powder, paprika, and basil to a shallow bowl or plate. Stir with a fork to combine.
2. In a separate shallow bowl, add the egg and whisk with a fork to combine.
3. Add the chicken to another plate and arrange the plates in the following order: chicken, egg, flour mixture, empty plate.

4. Dip each chicken piece into beaten egg with one hand, then with the other hand, dip the chicken into the flour mixture and pat the mixture onto the chicken to form an even coating.
5. Place the breaded chicken onto the empty fourth plate. Repeat with all the chicken pieces.
6. Heat a large skillet over medium heat. Add the oil, butter, and garlic. Cook for 30 seconds to a minute, just until the garlic is fragrant. Working in batches so as not to crowd the skillet, add the chicken and cook 4 to 5 minutes or until golden brown. Flip the chicken and cook an additional 3 to 4 minutes or until the chicken is cooked through and no longer pink in the center.

Recipe yields: 4 servings

Tofu and Broccoli with Yummy Sesame Sauce

INGREDIENTS:

- ¾ cups uncooked brown rice
- 1 block tofu (14 ounces), extra firm, cut into ¾-inch cubes
- 2 tablespoons arrowroot powder
- 1 tablespoon sesame oil
- 1 head broccoli, florets only
- 2 green onions, chopped

Yummy Sesame Sauce
- 1 teaspoon garlic powder
- ½ teaspoon ground ginger
- ¼ cup low-sodium soy sauce or liquid aminos
- 1 tablespoon sesame oil
- 1 tablespoon date syrup**
- 1 teaspoon rice vinegar
- ½ teaspoon chili garlic sauce (optional)

INSTRUCTIONS:

1. Cook the brown rice according to the package instructions.
2. Add the tofu cubes and arrowroot powder to a small bowl. Toss the tofu to coat it with the arrowroot powder.
3. Make the sesame sauce by combining the garlic powder, ginger, soy sauce, sesame oil, date syrup, rice vinegar, and chili garlic sauce (if desired) in a small bowl. Whisk to mix well.

RECIPES

4. Heat a large pan over medium heat. Add the sesame oil and tofu. Cook the tofu, stirring frequently, until lightly browned.
5. While the tofu is cooking, steam the broccoli: Add an inch of water to a medium pot and bring it to a boil over high heat. Lower the heat to medium and add the broccoli florets. Cover the pot and allow to steam for 5 to 6 minutes.
6. Once the tofu is browned, pour the sesame sauce over the tofu, lower the heat to low, and simmer, stirring frequently, for about 5 minutes.
7. To serve, add ½ cup cooked rice to a bowl and top with 1 cup of steamed broccoli and 4–5 ounces of tofu with sauce. Garnish with green onion.

Recipe yields: 3 servings

Almond Crusted Salmon with Asparagus and Quinoa for One

INGREDIENTS:

- 1 cup quinoa
- 6 spears asparagus, ends removed
- 1 teaspoon garlic powder
- 1 teaspoon onion powder
- 1 teaspoon dried parsley
- ½ teaspoon black pepper
- ¼ teaspoon salt
- 1 tablespoon almond flour**
- 1 tablespoon extra-virgin olive oil
- 4 ounce wild-caught salmon filet, skin removed

INSTRUCTIONS:

1. Preheat the oven to 350 degrees and begin cooking the quinoa according to package directions.
2. When the oven is heated, line a baking sheet with parchment paper and bake the asparagus on the sheet for 12 to 15 minutes, until slightly tender.
3. Meanwhile, in a shallow dish, combine the garlic powder, onion powder, parsley, pepper, salt, and almond flour. Stir with a fork to mix.
4. Heat a small skillet over medium heat. Add the oil.

5. Place the salmon in the dish with the seasonings and flour and turn the filet to coat it. Once it is coated, lightly tap any excess off.
6. Once the oil in the skillet is shimmering, add the salmon. Cook 3 to 4 minutes on the first side, until browned, then carefully flip and cook the other side for another 3 to 4 minutes, or until desired doneness. Salmon is done when you scrape the meat with a fork and it flakes easily.
7. Remove the asparagus from the oven and serve the salmon and asparagus with the cooked quinoa.

Recipe yields: 1 serving

Glass Noodle Lo Mein

INGREDIENTS:

- 2 packages (7.5 ounces each) sweet potato glass noodles
- 1 tablespoon avocado oil
- 1 pound protein of choice (tofu, chicken, shrimp, etc.), thinly sliced
- 1 zucchini, julienned
- 1 yellow squash, julienned
- ½ pound mushrooms, diced
- 1 small yellow onion, diced
- 3 green onions, chopped
- 2 cups kale, shredded
- 1 cup bok choy or napa cabbage, shredded
- 2 bell peppers, julienned
- 2 large carrots, julienned
- ½ cup water chestnuts drained and chopped (optional)
- 2 tablespoons low-sodium soy sauce
- ⅓ cup liquid aminos
- 1 tablespoon toasted sesame oil
- 1 tablespoon date syrup**
- 1 clove garlic, minced
- 1 inch ginger root, peeled and minced

INSTRUCTIONS:

1. Cook the glass noodles according to the package instructions.
2. Heat a large pan or wok over medium-high heat. Add the avocado oil. Once the oil is shimmering, add the protein.

Cook, stirring until browned and internal temperature reads 165 degrees. Remove the protein to a clean plate.
3. To the same pan, add the zucchini, squash, mushroom, yellow onion, kale, bok choy, bell peppers, carrot, and water chestnuts. Cook, stirring frequently, until the vegetables are crisp-tender, 3 to 4 minutes.
4. In a small bowl, combine the soy sauce, liquid aminos, sesame oil, date syrup, garlic, and ginger. Stir with a fork or whisk to mix.
5. Lower the heat to medium-low. Add the chicken back to the pan along with the cooked glass noodles. Pour the sauce over top and stir to coat evenly. Garnish with green onions and serve immediately.

Recipe yields: 4 servings

Creamy Spinach and Mushroom Pasta with Chicken

INGREDIENTS:

- 1 pound chickpea pasta or almond flour pasta, uncooked
- 1 tablespoon olive oil
- 4 cloves garlic, minced
- 1 pound chicken breast, thinly sliced, or chicken tenders
- 1 pound mushrooms, sliced
- 2 tablespoons butter
- ½ tablespoon almond flour**
- ¼ cup chicken or vegetable broth
- 1 cup heavy cream or dairy-free creamer (such as Nut Pods)
- ½ teaspoon Italian seasoning
- ½ cup parmesan cheese, grated
- 4 cups baby spinach
- 1 pinch salt
- ¼ teaspoon black pepper

INSTRUCTIONS:

1. Cook the pasta al dente according to the package instructions. Reserve ½ cup of pasta water.
2. Heat a large pan over medium heat. Add the oil and garlic and cook until the garlic is fragrant, about 1 minute.
3. Add the chicken and mushrooms and cook, stirring, until the chicken is browned and the internal temperature reads

165 degrees, about 7 minutes. Remove the chicken and mushrooms to a plate and keep warm.

4. Melt the butter in the same pan over medium-high heat. Whisk in the almond flour and cook for about a minute, whisking constantly.
5. Add the broth to the pan, whisking until smooth. Then lower the heat and simmer until the mixture is reduced, about 1 minute.
6. Add the cream, Italian seasoning, and parmesan cheese to the pan and whisk to incorporate. Then remove the pan from heat and add the spinach and ¼ cup of the reserved pasta water. Finally, add the cooked pasta, chicken, and mushrooms. Stir to combine and coat the pasta in sauce. Add more pasta water if needed to thin the sauce.
7. Season to taste with salt and pepper. Serve immediately.

Recipe yields: 4 servings

Dr. Rhona's Favorite One-Pan Tofu and Veggie Dinner

INGREDIENTS:

- 3 tablespoons olive oil
- 2 tablespoons lemon juice
- 2 tablespoons dried parsley
- ½ teaspoon cumin
- 1 teaspoon dried oregano
- 1 teaspoon dried dill weed
- 1 teaspoon paprika
- 1 teaspoon salt
- Pinch of black pepper
- Pinch of cayenne pepper
- 1 (14-ounce) block tofu, extra firm, cut into bite-size pieces

All chopped into bite-size pieces:
- 1 cup broccoli
- 1 cup red bell pepper
- 1 cup carrots
- 1 cup mushrooms
- 1 cup zucchini
- 1 cup red onion
- 1 cup tomato
- 2 shallots

INSTRUCTIONS:

1. Preheat the oven to 375 degrees. Line a baking sheet with parchment paper.
2. Meanwhile, in a small bowl, combine the oil, lemon juice, parsley, cumin, oregano, dill, paprika, salt, black pepper, and cayenne pepper. Whisk to mix well.

RECIPES

3. When the oven is heated, add the tofu, broccoli, bell pepper, carrot, mushroom, zucchini, onion, tomato, and shallots to the baking sheet. Pour the sauce over the tofu and vegetables and stir with a spatula to coat them.
4. Bake the tofu and veggies for 25 minutes, stirring occasionally.

Recipe yields: 3 servings

Quinoa Black Bean Burgers

INGREDIENTS:

- ¼ cup cooked quinoa
- 1 (15-ounce) can black beans, drained and rinsed
- ⅓ cup sun-dried tomatoes, diced
- ½ cup vegetable broth
- 6 tablespoons tomato paste
- 3 green onions, chopped
- 1 tablespoon olive oil
- 1 tablespoon smoked paprika
- ½ tablespoon garlic powder
- ½ tablespoon onion powder
- 1 teaspoon dried oregano
- 1 teaspoon dried parsley
- ¼ teaspoon salt
- ½ teaspoon black pepper

INSTRUCTIONS:

1. Preheat the oven to 400 degrees. Line a baking sheet with parchment paper.
2. Place the black beans into a large bowl and use a fork or potato masher to mash them.
3. Add the cooked quinoa, tomatoes, broth, tomato paste, onion, oil, paprika, garlic powder, onion powder, oregano, parsley, salt, and pepper. Stir with a spatula to combine.
4. Once thoroughly combined, the mixture will become thick. Scoop out 4 tablespoons of mixture to form each burger patty.

RECIPES

5. Place the patties on the baking sheet and bake for about 15 minutes or until lightly browned and heated through. Serve with your favorite vegetable and complex carbohydrate.

Recipe yields: 4 burgers (single serving size: 2 burgers)

Single Pan Roasted Chicken and Vegetables

INGREDIENTS:

- 1 teaspoon garlic powder
- 1 teaspoon onion powder
- ½ teaspoon black pepper
- ¼ teaspoon salt
- 1 teaspoon dried rosemary
- 1 teaspoon paprika
- 4 ounces boneless, skinless chicken breast
- 1 small russet potato, washed and chopped into ½-inch pieces
- ½ large red onion, chopped into ½-inch pieces
- ½ cup broccoli florets, chopped into ½-inch pieces
- ½ large carrot, chopped into ½-inch pieces
- 1 tablespoon extra-virgin olive oil

INSTRUCTIONS:

1. Preheat the oven to 350 degrees. In a small bowl, combine the garlic powder, onion powder, pepper, salt, rosemary, and paprika. Mix and set aside.
2. Place the chicken, potato, onion, broccoli, and carrot on a large baking sheet. Drizzle with the oil and sprinkle with the seasoning mix. Mix with hands until the chicken and vegetables are evenly coated.

RECIPES

3. Bake for 20 to 30 minutes, until the vegetables are starting to brown and the chicken's internal temperature measures 165 degrees.

Recipe yields: 1 serving

Turkey Taco Bowl

INGREDIENTS:

- ¼ cup uncooked brown rice
- ¼ teaspoon cumin
- ¼ teaspoon paprika
- ¼ teaspoon chili powder
- ¼ teaspoon oregano
- ¼ teaspoon garlic powder
- ¼ teaspoon onion powder
- ½ large white onion, chopped
- 1 bell pepper, chopped
- 4 teaspoons olive oil, divided
- 4 ounces 93%-lean ground turkey
- 1 tablespoon cheese of your choice, shredded
- 1 tablespoon full-fat, plain Greek yogurt
- 1 tablespoon salsa, without sugar
- 2 lettuce leaves, shredded

INSTRUCTIONS:

1. Preheat the oven to 425 degrees. Lightly grease a baking sheet and set aside.
2. Cook the brown rice according to the package instructions.
3. In a small bowl, make the taco seasoning mix by combining the cumin, paprika, chili powder, oregano, garlic powder, and onion powder. Mix with a fork. Set aside.
4. Spread the chopped onion and bell pepper on the baking sheet. Drizzle with 1 teaspoon olive oil, then bake the vegetables for 15 minutes, or until slightly golden brown.

RECIPES

5. While the vegetables are roasting, make the taco meat. Heat a large skillet over medium heat and add the oil. Once the oil is shimmering, add the ground turkey meat; cook until the meat is browned and reaches an internal temperature of 165 degrees.
6. Add the seasoning mix to the turkey. Stir to combine and simmer for 5 minutes.
7. Assemble the taco bowl by layering rice, turkey, roasted onion and pepper, shredded cheese, Greek yogurt, salsa, and lettuce.

Recipe yields: 1 serving

Simple Supper for One

INGREDIENTS:

- 1 medium (3 ounce) sweet potato, washed
- 1 tablespoon olive oil, plus extra if needed
- 4 ounces boneless, skinless chicken breast
- 2 cups broccoli florets
- 1 garlic clove, minced
- Pinch of salt
- Pinch of black pepper
- 2 tablespoons water

INSTRUCTIONS:

1. Prick the sweet potato all over with a fork, then microwave for 4 minutes, flipping halfway through. Cook for an additional 4 minutes, until the potato is thoroughly cooked.
2. While the potato is cooking, cook the chicken and broccoli. Heat a large skillet over medium heat and add the oil. Season the chicken with salt and pepper. Once the oil is shimmering, add the chicken and cook for about 7 minutes on each side, until the internal temperature reaches 165 degrees. Remove the chicken to a clean plate and set aside.
3. Lower the heat to medium-low. Add the broccoli and garlic to the skillet and additional oil if needed to keep the garlic from burning. Season with salt and pepper and

sauté the broccoli for 3 to 4 minutes. Add the water to the pan, cover, and cook until the broccoli is tender, 2 to 4 more minutes.

Recipe yields: 1 serving

SIDE DISH RECIPES

Green Beans with Almonds

INGREDIENTS:

- 1 tablespoon olive oil
- ½ cup slivered almonds
- 1 tablespoon butter
- 1 tablespoon minced garlic
- 1 pound green beans, washed, dried, and ends trimmed
- ¼ teaspoon salt
- ¼ teaspoon black pepper

INSTRUCTIONS:

1. Heat a large pan over low heat. Add the oil and slivered almonds. Cook, stirring, 2 to 3 minutes, until the almonds are golden brown. Remove the almonds from the pan and set them aside.
2. Add the butter and garlic to the pan and sauté for 1 minute.
3. Increase the heat to medium-high. Add the green beans and cook until crisp-tender, 4 to 5 minutes. Then add the almonds back to the pan. Remove from heat and season to taste with salt and pepper. Serve immediately.

Recipe yields: 2 servings

Mushroom Soup

INGREDIENTS:

- 2 tablespoons olive oil
- 4 shallots, chopped
- 1½ pounds cremini mushrooms, washed and dried, stems removed, chopped
- 1½ pounds portobello mushrooms, washed and dried, stems removed, chopped
- 1 teaspoon salt, and more if needed
- ¼ cup sherry wine** or DIY substitute (see below)
- ½ cup oat flour or almond flour**
- 4 cups low-sodium vegetable stock
- Pinch of black pepper

INSTRUCTIONS:

1. Heat a 4-quart soup pot over medium heat. Add the oil, shallots, mushrooms, and salt. Sauté the vegetables and allow to sweat for about 10 minutes or until vegetables are tender.
2. Add the sherry wine and continue to cook until the liquid has almost evaporated. Add in the flour and stir for 5 minutes to cook the flour.
3. Add the vegetable stock to the pot while whisking the vegetables and broth. Increase heat to high until the soup

begins to boil. Reduce the heat to medium-low and let the soup simmer, with the lid ajar, for about 30 minutes.
4. Add the black pepper and more salt if needed. Remove the pot from the heat and allow the soup to cool slightly, then use an immersion blender to puree until creamy. Serve warm.

DIY Sherry Wine Substitute:
- ⅓ cup water
- ⅓ cup unsweetened apple juice
- 3 tablespoons apple cider vinegar
- ¼ teaspoon low-sodium soy sauce or liquid aminos

Combine water, apple juice, vinegar, and soy sauce in a small bowl or jar. Mix and use in recipes that call for sherry cooking wine.

Note: Sherry contains 4g of sugar in the form of carbohydrate and could be a trigger. Omit from the recipe if you want to stay on the safe side.

Recipe yields: 8 servings (single serving size: 1 cup)

Everyone Loves This Grilled Broccoli (Even Kids!)

INGREDIENTS:

- 1 pound broccoli florets, washed and trimmed
- 8 garlic cloves, peeled and left whole
- 3 tablespoons olive oil
- Pinch of salt
- Pinch of black pepper

INSTRUCTIONS:

1. Add the broccoli, garlic, oil, salt, and pepper to a large bowl. Toss to combine.
2. Heat a grill pan (one with ridges) at medium heat on the stovetop, then add the broccoli mixture. Cook for about 10 minutes, or until the garlic and broccoli begin to char. Serve immediately.

Recipe yields: 2 servings

Dr. Rhona's Favorite Brussels Sprouts

INGREDIENTS:

- 1 pound Brussels sprouts, trimmed and cut in half
- 1 tablespoon olive oil
- 1 teaspoon salt
- 1 teaspoon black pepper
- 1 teaspoon garlic powder
- Sprinkle of parmesan cheese

INSTRUCTIONS:

1. Preheat the oven to 400 degrees, and line a baking sheet with parchment paper.
2. Add the Brussels sprouts to the baking sheet. Drizzle with the oil, and sprinkle with the salt, pepper, and garlic powder. Toss with tongs or hands to evenly coat the sprouts.
3. Roast for about 20 minutes, tossing after 10 minutes. Just as the sprouts are browning at the edges, add parmesan cheese for the last minute of cooking.

Recipe yields: 2 servings

RECIPES

Vegetable Stir-Fry with Rice for One

INGREDIENTS:

- ¼ cup uncooked brown rice
- 1 tablespoon olive oil
- 4 ounces chicken breast, cut into 1-inch pieces
- 2 cups mixed vegetables (consider broccoli, bell peppers, carrots, cabbage, and/or onions)
- ¼ teaspoon garlic powder
- ¼ teaspoon ginger powder
- ¼ teaspoon onion powder
- 2 tablespoons low-sodium soy sauce or liquid aminos
- ¼ teaspoon sesame oil

INSTRUCTIONS:

1. Cook the brown rice according to package directions.
2. Preheat a large skillet over medium-high heat and add the oil. Add the chicken breast and sauté until browned and internal temperature reads 165 degrees. Remove the chicken to a clean plate.
3. Add the vegetables to the skillet and cook for 10 minutes, until al dente.
4. In a small bowl, combine the garlic powder, ginger powder, onion powder, soy sauce, and sesame oil. Whisk to mix well.
5. Return the chicken to the skillet and add the sauce. Cook 2 to 3 minutes until the sauce is bubbly.
6. Remove from heat and serve over the brown rice.

Recipe yields: 1 serving

DRESSING RECIPES

Bright Citrus Dressing

INGREDIENTS:

- 1 lime
- 1 orange
- 1 tablespoon Dijon mustard
- 3 tablespoons olive oil
- 1 cup fresh basil leaves, finely chopped
- Pinch of salt
- Pinch of black pepper
- 1 tablespoon sesame or poppy seeds** (optional)

INSTRUCTIONS:

1. First, zest the lime and set aside. Then cut the lime in half and squeeze for 2 tablespoons of juice. Do the same for the orange, collecting zest and 4 tablespoons of juice.
2. In a small bowl, combine the lime zest, lime juice, orange zest, orange juice, mustard, oil, basil, salt, pepper, and seeds if desired. Whisk to combine.
3. Use immediately or store in an airtight container in the refrigerator for up to 5 days. Measure and add the remaining ingredients, stirring well to combine.

Recipe yields: 12 servings (single serving size: 1 tablespoon)

Ginger Peanut Dressing

INGREDIENTS:

- 1 teaspoon ginger root, grated
- 1 teaspoon garlic, minced
- 2 tablespoons unsweetened peanut butter
- 1 tablespoon low-sodium soy sauce or liquid aminos
- 1 tablespoon sesame oil
- 1 lime, juiced (about 2 tablespoons)
- 1 to 2 tablespoons water, divided

INSTRUCTIONS:

1. In a small bowl or jar, combine the ginger, garlic, peanut butter, soy sauce, sesame oil, lime juice, and 1 tablespoon of water. Stir with a fork or small whisk to combine.
2. At first the peanut butter will separate when it comes into contact with the water, lime, and soy sauce. Just continue stirring until smooth. If the dressing is too thick, add more water and stir to thin.
3. Use immediately or store in an airtight container in the refrigerator for up to 5 days.

Recipe yields: 10 servings (single serving size: 1 tablespoon)

Herbed Tahini Dressing

INGREDIENTS:

- 2 lemons
- ½ cup tahini
- ¼ cup plus 2 tablespoons cold water, and more if needed
- 2 tablespoons olive oil
- 2 cloves garlic, minced
- ¼ cup fresh parsley leaves
- ¼ cup fresh cilantro leaves
- ¼ cup fresh chives
- ¼ teaspoon salt, and more if needed

INSTRUCTIONS:

1. First, zest one lemon to create 2 teaspoons zest. Then cut both lemons in half and squeeze, to create ¼ cup lemon juice.
2. Add all the following ingredients into a blender, food processor, or the cup of an immersion blender: lemon zest, lemon juice, tahini, water, and oil. Blend until just combined. Add the garlic, parsley, cilantro, chives, and salt and blend until smooth. Taste and add more salt if needed. If the dressing seems too thick, add a bit more water.
3. Use immediately or store in an airtight container in the refrigerator for up to 5 days. This dressing makes a great snack when paired with raw veggies.

Recipe yields: 16 servings (single serving size: 1 tablespoon)

SNACK RECIPES

Toasted Oats

INGREDIENTS:

- ½ cup old-fashioned rolled oats
- 2 teaspoons coconut oil
- 1 tablespoon unsweetened coconut
- ¼ teaspoon ground cinnamon
- 1 teaspoon butter, melted

INSTRUCTIONS:

1. Add the oats, coconut oil, coconut, cinnamon, and melted butter to a small bowl. Stir to combine.
2. Place the mixture into a large skillet and slowly heat on the stove over medium-low heat until the mixture becomes a light brown color, or place in a 300-degree oven on a lined baking sheet and bake for 10 to 20 minutes (until the mixture is lightly toasted).

These oats are great with milk or yogurt and fruit.

Recipe yields: 1 serving

Kickin' Chickpeas

INGREDIENTS:

- 1 (15 ounce) can of chickpeas, drained, then rinsed and dried
- 1 tablespoon olive oil
- 1 teaspoon salt
- 1 teaspoon black pepper
- 1 teaspoon paprika
- 1 teaspoon chili powder
- 1 teaspoon onion powder
- 1 teaspoon garlic powder

INSTRUCTIONS:

1. Preheat the oven to 350 degrees. Line a baking sheet with parchment paper.
2. Add the chickpeas to a medium bowl with the oil, salt, pepper, paprika, chili powder, onion powder, and garlic powder. Stir with a spatula to evenly distribute the oil and seasoning mixture. Spread the chickpeas on the baking sheet.
3. Bake for 25 minutes, stirring frequently, until the chickpeas are crisp. Allow to cool, then use in salads or as a crunchy snack. These are best eaten quickly; they lose their crispiness as time goes on. Store in a loosely covered container at room temperature for about five days (refrigerating them will make them chewy).

Recipe yields: 4 servings

Cinnamon Banana Nice-Cream

INGREDIENTS:

- 4 bananas, peeled, mashed, frozen, and slightly defrosted
- 4 tablespoons unsweetened milk of choice
- ¼ teaspoon cinnamon
- ½ teaspoon vanilla extract

INSTRUCTIONS:

1. Add the bananas, milk, cinnamon, and vanilla to a blender, and blend until smooth.
2. Place the nice-cream into a freezer-safe container and freeze for 1 to 2 hours until firm. Scoop as you would ice cream.

Recipe yields: 4 servings

HOLIDAY RECIPES

Unsweetened Pumpkin Spice Breakfast Cookies

INGREDIENTS:

- 4 ripe bananas, peeled and mashed
- ½ cup unsweetened organic canned pumpkin
- ½ cup unsweetened applesauce
- ¾ cup frozen blueberries
- 1 tablespoon pumpkin spice seasoning
- 4 cups organic rolled oats
- 2 tablespoons unsweetened almond butter**

INSTRUCTIONS:

1. Preheat oven to 400 degrees. Line a baking sheet with parchment paper.
2. In a large bowl, combine the bananas, pumpkin, applesauce, blueberries, pumpkin spice, oats, and almond butter. Stir with a spatula until incorporated.
3. For each cookie, scoop 2 tablespoons of the dough and flatten it into a circle, placing each 1 inch apart on the baking sheet.

4. Bake for 20 minutes, until the cookies are slightly golden brown. The cookies will only expand slightly during baking.

Note: Mix up the flavors in this cookie by adding a shot of vanilla cream stevia** to the dough. Or make an apple cinnamon version by omitting the pumpkin and pumpkin spice and using an extra ½ cup unsweetened applesauce and 1 tablespoon of cinnamon.

Recipe yields: 24 cookies (single serving size: 2 cookies)

Pork Tenderloin with Sprouts and Squash

INGREDIENTS:

- 1 tablespoon garlic powder
- 1 tablespoon onion powder
- 1 tablespoon cumin
- 1 tablespoon chili powder
- ½ tablespoon black pepper
- ½ tablespoon paprika
- ¾ teaspoon salt
- 2 pounds pork tenderloin
- 2 tablespoons extra-virgin olive oil, divided
- 2 pounds butternut squash, chopped
- 2 pounds Brussels sprouts, each cut in half
- ½ lemon, juiced

INSTRUCTIONS:

1. Preheat the oven to 400 degrees.
2. In a small bowl, combine the garlic powder, onion powder, cumin, chili powder, pepper, paprika, and salt. Stir with a fork to mix.
3. Place the pork tenderloin onto one side of a baking sheet and drizzle with 1 tablespoon of the oil. Sprinkle with the spice blend and rub the seasoning onto the pork to create an even coating.
4. Place the pork into the oven and bake for 30 minutes.

5. Remove the baking sheet and add the squash and Brussels sprouts to the other side of the baking sheet. Drizzle the vegetables with the other 1 tablespoon oil and stir to coat.
6. Return the pan to the oven and bake for 5 to 10 minutes or until the squash and sprouts are browning and the pork has reached an internal temperature of 145 degrees. Squeeze lemon juice over the pork before serving.

Recipe yields: 8 servings

Party Pleasing Apple and Pear Crisp

INGREDIENTS:

Filling
- 1 tablespoon coconut oil, melted
- 1 pound Granny Smith or Jonagold apples, cored, peeled, and thinly sliced
- 1 pound D'Anjou or Bartlett pears, cored, peeled, and thinly sliced
- 1 tablespoon lemon juice
- ¼ cup date syrup**
- 1 teaspoon vanilla extract
- 1 tablespoon arrowroot powder
- 1 teaspoon cinnamon
- ½ teaspoon sea salt
- ½ cup unsweetened apple juice

Topping
- 1½ cups rolled oats
- ½ cup almond flour**
- ½ cup walnuts or pecans, coarsely chopped
- Pinch of sea salt
- 1 tablespoon cinnamon
- ⅓ cup date syrup**
- ¼ cup unsweetened applesauce or ¼ cup coconut oil

INSTRUCTIONS:

1. Preheat the oven to 400 degrees. Use the coconut oil to lightly grease the bottom and sides of a 2-quart baking dish. Add the sliced apples and pears and set to the side.

RECIPES

2. In a small bowl, combine the lemon juice, date syrup, vanilla, arrowroot powder, cinnamon, salt, and apple juice. Stir until mixed well and no clumps of arrowroot powder remain. Pour the mixture over the apples and pears. Toss the fruit to coat it evenly with the syrup.
3. For the topping, stir the oats, almond flour, nuts, salt, and cinnamon together in a medium bowl. Add the date syrup and applesauce to the mixture and stir with a fork until small, sticky crumbs form. Spread the topping evenly over the fruit.
4. Cover the dish and bake for 45 minutes, until the fruit is bubbling and has softened. Remove the cover and bake for an additional 15 minutes until the topping is golden brown.

Recipe yields: 12 servings (single serving size: ½ cup)

DR. RHONA'S FOOD FREEDOM TIPS

We've created this handy checklist for you take a picture of or scan and print, so you can have it at your desk, in your cupboard, at work—wherever you'll see it often—so you can remind yourself daily of how to stay free from food chaos.

1. **Always put recovery first!** When food is in its right place, there is freedom to live without food chatter and chaos.
2. **Plan ahead.** Make a plan for your meals and stick to it. It doesn't have to be perfect, as long as it's nourishing and satisfying. Remember: if you fail to plan, you plan to fail.
3. **Prepare.** Stock up at the grocery store weekly with all you need to stick to your satisfying and nourishing food plan. Take time each week to prepare for success. Find (or create) shortcuts that make it easy to stick to your plan.
4. **Think ahead.** What is your day going to be like? Your week? Will there be days when you need to make your meals ahead of time because you'll be out and about? Don't wait until you're running

from appointment to appointment and are stuck on the road without what you need.

5. **Be mindful!** Every day, take time to reflect on something to help you remember your recovery mindset. Use recovery readings, meetings, phone calls, texts, etc., so you don't forget. Amnesia sets in quicker than you think. Practice the 12 Steps. They work!

6. **Clean your mental mess every day.** Built-up stress and untended emotions are two of the biggest triggers for food abuse. Pay attention. Use a feelings list or journal. Call a friend who understands. Talk to God on a prayer walk. Don't ignore your feelings. They need some love and attention.

7. **Spirituality is key.** Fill up on what your heart really needs. Take time every day to breathe, rest, meditate, and pray. Learn to live in peace. God's love fills the place where food once was. Let His love fill you up. Let Him comfort you.

8. **Rely on support.** Have a posse of at least five people you can call or text for encouragement, truth, butt-kicking, love, comfort, prayer, and

help in sorting out complicated stuff. Supportive people can be so much more helpful than ice cream and cookies.

9. **Be clear about your food boundaries.** Learn your lines and stick to them. Clarify what foods and food behaviors trigger addictive eating and insanity for you, and avoid them.

10. **Believe!** All things are possible with God. Never give up. The battle is real, but you can recover. Take it one day at a time and keep moving forward in faith. Who the Son sets free *is* free indeed (John 8:36).

ACKNOWLEDGMENTS

There are many people without whom this book would not have been possible, and I owe them many thanks.

Matt West: for being a great leader of the Dexterity team, a supportive friend, and a wise guide. Kim West: for managing the business aspects of all things Dexterity. Ashley Harris: for support through the years in marketing the *Satisfied* brand. Jocelyn Bailey: for super helpful editing and overall wise and sensible writing direction (and such a pleasure to work with to boot!). Jessie Epstein: for your exceptional writing talent and incredible work ethic; you are an amazing team player and you did a great job of capturing my voice and putting the words together in style. Danielle Ruditsky: for your social media expertise and being our number-one cheerleader; thank you for keeping the *Satisfied* brand out there so people can get the help we have to offer. Joel Ruditsky: for your support, encouragement, and insight. Robert Staffa: for your patience, support, and love, as well as video and graphic design help.

Special thanks to my clients, past and present, as well as *Satisfied Experience* group members: so much of what I know comes from our honest and authentic journeys to food freedom together. Big thanks to my AACC companions, particularly Tim Clinton and Jennifer Cisney Ellers: thank you for believing in biblically based food addiction recovery, and for a faith-based platform to provide help to people everywhere. Jackie Mack: thank you for your incredible dietary guidelines, suggestions, and recipes, and for helping so many of our mutual clients and *Satisfied Experience* members. You are a blessing to all the people you are helping find food freedom!

David Wiss: thank you for your gracious, thorough, and excellent editorial review. Your contribution was invaluable.

My deepest gratitude to so many professionals, researchers, and champions—too many to name—who have helped bring validation to the science behind sugar and processed food addiction.

Most of all, I'd like to acknowledge and thank the people in recovery who are living proof that sugar and processed food addiction is real and recovery is possible.

And finally, I thank God Almighty for my freedom from addictive eating and obsessive thinking about food and weight for decades, and for the ability to pass it on to bring healing to others.

APPENDIX
Additional Food Plans

ACTIVE LIFESTYLES

More than ever, active individuals typically do some form of higher-intensity workouts such as distance running or hour-long classes. This is different from going up and down stairs at work, walking the dog, or the occasional trip to the gym. If *active* describes you, that means you should consume more protein, especially on the days you exercise. It's how you properly fuel your body for workouts. Making sure you eat enough protein keeps you full and satisfied throughout the day, meaning less opportunity for confusion and triggers.

A high-protein snack could be a cup of yogurt with six ounces of fruit, or a cheese stick and a hard-boiled egg, or six ounces of strawberries with an eight-ounce glass of milk.

If you're looking to have fewer snacks and focus on protein in your meals, that could look like eggs for breakfast, a salmon quinoa bowl for lunch, and chicken and stir-fried vegetables for dinner. We want to make sure that you are satisfied, that you're avoiding haphazard eating, and that your body is getting the nutrients it needs to perform. Take a look at the options below to determine which plan might be right for you.

ADDITIONAL FOOD PLANS

Plan E

PLAN

Breakfast:
Protein: 3 oz Women, 4 oz Men
Carbohydrate: 1 oz
Fruit: 6 oz
Healthy fat: 1 tbsp or 0.5 oz
Dairy: 1 c or 8 oz

Lunch:
Protein: 3 oz Women, 4 oz Men
Carbohydrate: 2 oz
Vegetable: 2–3 c raw or 1–2 c cooked
Healthy fat: 1 tbsp or 0.5 oz
Fruit: 6 oz

Dinner:
Protein: 3 oz Women, 4 oz Men
Carbohydrate: ½–1 c
Vegetable: 2–3 c raw or 1–2 c cooked
Healthy fat: 1 tbsp or 0.5 oz

SAMPLE

Eggs & Yogurt Parfait:
Eggs: 3–4 eggs
Toasted oats: 1 oz
Blackberries: 6 oz
Olive oil: 1 tbsp or 0.5 oz
Yogurt: 8 oz

Grilled Chicken Wrap:
Chicken: 3 oz Women, 4 oz Men
**1 Ezekiel wrap
Salad greens: 2–3 c raw or 1–2 c cooked
Avocado or dressing: 1 tbsp or 0.5 oz
Pear: 6 oz

Tofu & Broccoli w/ Yummy Sesame Sauce:
Tofu: 3 oz Women, 4 oz Men
Brown rice: ½–1 c
Broccoli: 2–3 c raw or 1–2 c cooked
**Sesame seeds: ½ tbsp or 0.5 oz
Sesame oil: ½ tbsp or 0/5 oz

For more active people, this is an option to focus on more protein while avoiding the need for snacks in between. The protein will keep you satiated while keeping you on the move.

Plan F

PLAN

Breakfast:
Carbohydrate: 1 oz
Healthy fat: 1 tbsp or 0.5 oz
Dairy: 1 c or 8 oz
Fruit: 6 oz

Snack:
Protein: 1 oz
Fruit: 6 oz

Lunch:
Protein: 3 oz Women, 4 oz Men
Carbohydrate: ½–1 c
Vegetable: 2–3 c raw or 1–2 c cooked
Healthy fat: 1 tbsp or 0.5 oz

Dinner:
Protein: 3 oz Women, 4 oz Men
Carbohydrate: 3 oz
Vegetable: 2–3 c raw 1–2 c cooked
Healthy fat: 2 tbsp or 1 oz

SAMPLE

Yogurt & Toasted Oats:
Toasted oats: 1 oz
**Walnuts: 1 tbsp or 0.5 oz
Yogurt: 1 c or 8 oz
Apple: 6 oz

Fruit & Cheese:
Cheese stick: 1 oz
Apple: 6 oz

Shrimp & Veggies:
Shrimp: 3 oz Women, 4 oz Men
Brown rice: ½–1 c
Bell peppers & onions: 2–3 c raw or 1–2 c cooked
Olive oil: 1 tbsp or 0.5 oz

Chicken & Sprouts:
Chicken: 3 oz Women, 4 oz Men
Potatoes: 3 oz
Brussels sprouts: 1–2 c cooked
Olive oil: 2 tbsp or 1 oz

If you want to eat three meals with an additional protein-packed snack, this is the right choice for you. This plan promotes consistent blood sugar levels post-workout.

ADDITIONAL FOOD PLANS

Plan G

PLAN

Breakfast:
Protein: 2 oz women, 3 oz men
Carbohydrate: 1 oz
Healthy fat: 1 tbsp or 0.5 oz
Fruit: 6 oz

Snack:
Protein: 1 oz
Fruit: 6 oz

Lunch:
Protein: 3 oz Women, 4 oz Men
Vegetable: 2–3 c raw or 1–2 c cooked
Healthy Fat: 1 tbsp or 0.5 oz

Snack:
Dairy: 1 c or 8 oz
Carbohydrate: 1 oz

Dinner:
Protein: 3 oz Women, 4 oz Men
Carbohydrate: 3 oz
Vegetable: 2–3 c raw or 1–2 c cooked
Healthy fat: 2 tbsp or 1 oz

SAMPLE

Eggs & Toast:
Eggs: 2–3 eggs
**Ezekiel bread: 1 oz
Butter: 1 tbsp or 0.5 oz
Cantaloupe: 6 oz

Protein Pick-Me-Up:
Cheese stick: 1 oz
Orange: 6 oz

Tuna on a Salad:
Tuna: 3 oz Women, 4 oz Men
Salad greens: 2–3 c raw or 1–2 c cooked
Dressing: 1 tbsp or 0.5 oz

Yogurt & Toasted Oats:
Yogurt: 1 c or 8 oz
Toasted oats: 1 oz

Chicken, Sweet Potato, & Cauliflower:
Chicken: 3 oz Women, 4 oz Men
Sweet potato: 3 oz
Cauliflower: 1–2 c cooked
Butter: 2 tbsp or 1 oz

This plan is a great option if you are on the go all day long and need to keep your energy high.

Plan H

PLAN

Breakfast:
Protein: 2 oz Women, 3 oz Men
Vegetable: 2–3 c raw or 1–2 c cooked
Healthy fat: 1 tbsp or 0.5 oz
Fruit: 6 oz

Snack:
Protein: 1 oz
Fruit: 6 oz

Lunch:
Protein: 3 oz Women, 4 oz Men
Carbohydrate: ½–1 c
Vegetable: 2–3 c raw or 1–2 c cooked
Healthy fat: 1 tbsp or 0.5 oz

Snack:
Vegetable: 1–2 c raw or ½–1 c cooked
Healthy fat: 1 tbsp or 0.5 oz

Dinner:
Protein: 3 oz Women, 4 oz Men
Carbohydrate: 3 oz
Vegetable: 2–3 c raw or 1–2 c cooked
Healthy fat: 1 tbsp or 0.5 oz

Snack:
Dairy: 1 c or 8 oz
Fruit: 6 oz

SAMPLE

Veggie Omelet & Fruit:
Eggs: 2–3 eggs
Mixed veggies: 1–2 c cooked
Avocado: 1 tbsp or 0.5 oz
Blueberries: 6 oz

Plant Power:
Soy beans: 1 oz
Mandarin oranges: 6 oz

Salmon Grain Bowl:
Salmon: 3 oz Women, 4 oz Men
**Quinoa: ½–1 c
Eggplant: 1–2 c cooked
Olive oil: 1 tbsp or 0.5 oz

Veggie & Dip:
Carrots: 1–2 c raw
Guacamole: 1 tbsp or 0.5 oz

Roasted Turkey & Veggies:
Roasted turkey: 3 oz Women, 4 oz Men
Potatoes: 3 oz
Collard greens: 1–2 c cooked
Butter: 1 tbsp or 0.5 oz

Raspberries & Cream:
Milk: 1 c or 8 oz
Raspberries: 6 oz

Three meals and three snacks will give you the energy you need while avoiding that blood sugar rollercoaster, especially for highly active people.

NOTES

1. D. A. Wiss, N. Avena, and P. Rada, "Sugar Addiction: From Evolution to Revolution," *Frontiers in Psychiatry* 9 (2018): 545, https://doi.org/10.3389/fpsyt.2018.00545.
2. Wiss, Avena, and Rada, "Sugar Addiction." Dr. David Wiss has a wealth of research resources on this topic at www.wisemindnutrition.com.
3. S. H. Ahmed, K. Guillem, and Y. Vandaele, "Sugar Addiction: Pushing the Drug-Sugar Analogy to the Limit," *Current Opinion in Clinical Nutrition and Metabolic Care* 16, no. 4 (2013): 434–9, https://doi.org/10.1097/MCO.0b013e328361c8b8.
4. T. Peters et al., "The Association of Serum Leptin Levels with Food Addiction Is Moderated by Weight Status in Adolescent Psychiatric Inpatients," *European Eating Disorders Review: The Journal of the Eating Disorders Association* 26, no. 6 (2018): 618–28, https://doi.org/10.1002/erv.2637.
5. Y. Yu, R. Miller, and S. W. Groth, "A Literature Review of Dopamine in Binge Eating," *Journal of Eating Disorders* 10, no. 11 (2022), https://doi.org/10.1186/s40337-022-00531-y.
6. James Clear, "How Long Does It Actually Take to Form a New Habit? (Backed by Science)," February 4, 2020, jamesclear.com/new-habit.
7. Mark Hyman, MD, "10 Rules to Eat Safely for Life (and What to Remove from Your Kitchen)," February 2, 2012, https://drhyman.com/blogs/content/10-rules-to-eat-safely-for-life-and-what-to-remove-from-your-kitchen/.
8. Rhona Epstein, *Satisfied: A 90-Day Spiritual Journey Toward Food Freedom* (Nashville: Dexterity, 2018).

NOTES

9. Rhona Epstein, *The Satisfied Workbook: A Spiritual Guide to Recovery and Food Freedom* (Nashville: Dexterity, 2021).
10. James Clear, *Atomic Habits: Tiny Changes, Remarkable Results: An Easy and Proven Way to Build Good Habits and Break Bad Ones* (New York: Avery, 2022).
11. "Carbohydrates and Blood Sugar," Harvard T. H. Chan School of Public Health, May 9, 2024, https://nutritionsource.hsph.harvard.edu/carbohydrates/carbohydrates-and-blood-sugar/.
12. R. Ajmera, "Sweet Potato Glycemic Index: Boiled, Roasted, Baked, and Fried," Healthline, September 23, 2019, https://www.healthline.com/nutrition/sweet-potato-glycemic-index#bottom-line.
13. A. Abizaid and T. L. Horvath, "Ghrelin and the Central Regulation of Feeding and Energy Balance," *Indian Journal of Endocrinology and Metabolism* (16 December 2012), https://www.ncbi.nlm.nih.gov/pmc/articles/PMC3602992/.
14. R. Aylott and V. Mitchell, "An Exploratory Study of Grocery Shopping Stressors," *International Journal of Retail and Distribution Management* 26, no. 9 (1998): 362–73, https://doi.org/10.1108/09590559810237908.
15. A. W. K. Yeung, "Bibliometric Analysis on the Literature of Monk Fruit Extract and Mogrosides as Sweeteners," *Frontiers in Nutrition* (10 August 29, 2023), https://doi.org/10.3389/fnut.2023.1253255.
16. H. O. Mirghani, "Dates Fruits Effects on Blood Glucose Among Patients with Diabetes Mellitus: A Review and Meta-Analysis," *Pakistan Journal of Medical Sciences* (2021), https://doi.org/10.12669/pjms.37.4.4112.
17. "Does What You Eat Affect Your Mood?" January 12, 2021, Cleveland Clinic, https://health.clevelandclinic.org/bad-mood-look-to-your-food.
18. J. Firth et al., "Food and Mood: How Do Diet and Nutrition Affect Mental Wellbeing?" *BMJ* (June 29, 2020), https://doi.org/10.1136/bmj.m2382.

NOTES

19. Firth et al., "Food and Mood."
20. V. Vigar et al., "A Systematic Review of Organic Versus Conventional Food Consumption: Is There a Measurable Benefit on Human Health?" *Nutrients* (December 18, 2019), https://doi.org/10.3390/nu12010007.
21. Northwestern Medicine, "Celiac Disease vs. Gluten Intolerance," August 2019, https://www.nm.org/healthbeat/healthy-tips/celiac-disease-vs-gluten-intolerance-infographic.
22. Lisa Jahns, *Water: An Important Part of a Healthy Winter Diet*, Agricultural Research Service, United States Department of Agriculture, last updated September 11, 2023, https://www.ars.usda.gov/plains-area/gfnd/gfhnrc/docs/news-articles/2012/water-an-important-part-of-a-healthy-winter-diet/.
23. *Physical Activity Guidelines for Americans*, 2nd ed., US Department of Health and Human Services (2018), chrome-extension://efaidnbmnnnibpcajpcglclefindmkaj/https://health.gov/sites/default/files/2019-09/Physical_Activity_Guidelines_2nd_edition.pdf.

ABOUT THE AUTHORS

Rhona Epstein, PsyD, CAC, is a licensed psychologist, addictions counselor, and marriage and family therapist, as well as an award-winning author of multiple books on topics related to food addiction and recovery, including *Food Triggers*, *Satisfied*, and *The Satisfied Workbook*. She began her recovery journey as a teen after battling binge eating and bulimia from childhood.

Affected so deeply by the recovery process, she determined to devote the rest of her life to helping others climb out of the same insanity with food abuse and weight obsession. She completed a marriage and family therapy training program through the Council for Relationships at the University of Pennsylvania in 1988. Since 1994, Dr. Rhona has provided individual, couple, family, and group therapy and coaching online and in her private practice. She received her doctorate in clinical psychology from Chestnut Hill College in 2009.

Dr. Rhona calls the Philadelphia, Pennsylvania area home; *The Satisfied Guide to Eating Well* is her fifth book. To learn more, visit www.drrhona.com.

ABOUT THE AUTHORS

Jackie Mack, MS, RDN, LDN, is a dietician, farm keeper, and accidental entrepreneur. She graduated from West Chester University of Pennsylvania with a bachelor of science degree in nutrition and dietetics and a master of science degree in community nutrition. She currently resides in Montgomery County, Pennsylvania, with her goats, chickens, and loving husband. *The Satisfied Guide to Eating Well* is her first book.

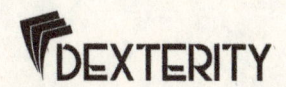

More Than 35,000 Copies Sold

"Dr. Rhona brings the wonderful worlds of science and faith together, to chart a brilliant path to freedom."
—DR. TOM CLINTON, President of the American Association of Christian Counselors

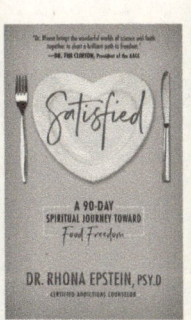

ISBN 9780998325323 • $15.99   ISBN 9781947297197 • $16.95   ISBN 9781947297678 • $16.95   ISBN 9781947297944 • $18.95

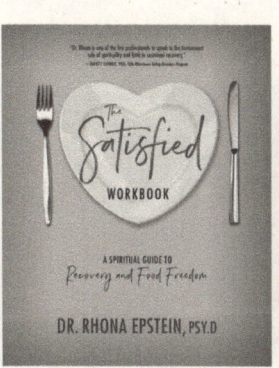

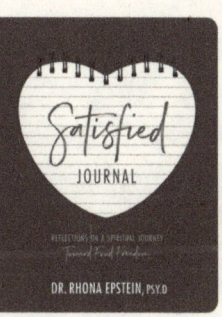

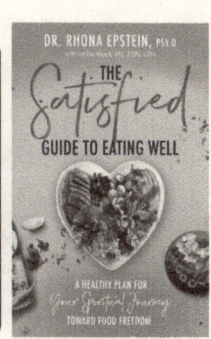

Visit DrRhona.com or DexterityBooks.com to order.

The Satisfied Experience: An Online Program with Dr. Rhona

For anyone who knows they need more than a diet to transform their relationship with food and overeating for good!

- Quit endless cycles of overeating, dieting & losing control with food
- Calm cravings for excess food
- Make peace with food and your body
- Group support

- Biblically based inspiration & hope
- Daily guidance through the 12 steps
- Daily prayers & meditations
- Weekly live coaching

Visit DrRhona.com and JMnutritionalcounseling.squarespace.com for more information
Follow Dr. Rhona and Jackie Mack on social media.

@DrRhona
@DrRhonaOfficial
@Dr.Rhona

@jmnutritionalcounseling
@JMNutritionalCounseling
@jmnutritionalcounseling

DEXTERITY

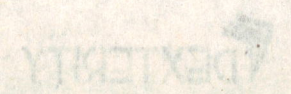